P9-AQL-558

NEITHER SAFE NOR EFFECTIVE

The Evidence Against
The COVID Vaccines

From

Government institutions

CDC
FDA
HHS
US Federal Court
GOV.UK
Public Health Scotland
Government of Denmark
Government of Canada

Medical journals

JAMA
NEJM
Nature
Vaccine
Journal of Pediatrics
Circulation
Pediatric Cardiology
Nature Microbiology

And Pfizer, Moderna and Walgreens

Dr. Colleen Huber

May 20, 2022

Dedication

This book is dedicated to Ernesto Ramirez, Jr. who lost his life, at 16 years old, just 5 days after his first Pfizer vaccine, an event verified on autopsy by four independent physicians, although Ernesto played sports and had no health problems before the vaccine.

This book is also dedicated to all those who lost loved ones following vaccines, or who tried to talk a loved one out of a vaccine, or who risked their source of income or their education, standing strong against peer pressure, bullying, superstition and "mandates."

Dedication

CONTENTS

NEITHER SAFE NOR EFFECTIVE:
The Evidence Against
The COVID Vaccines

© 2022 Dr. Colleen Huber NMD
Naturopathic Medical Doctor
Tempe, Arizona, USA

What do we know about the COVID vaccines?

What we knew by 2021

Chapter 1

Danger signals
from human and animal studies

I am a Naturopathic Medical Doctor in Arizona, and in this state I have served as a medical expert witness regarding vaccine injury and vaccine safety considerations in court cases. I ask that you, the reader, consider the information below, before submitting to the experimental COVID vaccine.

THIS CHAPTER IS A

BLACK BOX EMERGENCY DOCUMENT

The following outline is written with a lot of bold print, in case of an emergency need to get this information to a parent who is considering taking their children for the COVID vaccines. **These next several pages must be read first before an irreversible medical experiment is done.** The rest of this book painstakingly makes the case about hazards related to the COVID vaccines, through hundreds of scientific studies and government data pages, but this chapter is especially for emergency use.

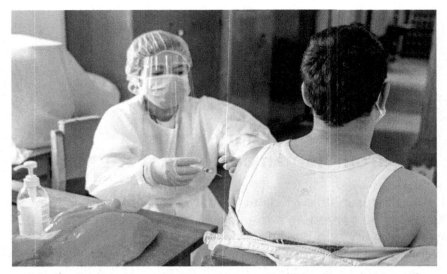

Injecting the brand-new substance. How much of this will people tolerate?

1) **Is the COVID vaccine experimental?** The FDA granted emergency use authorization for these vaccines. [1] Emergency use authorization is permitted by law *only* if there are no effective treatments for COVID. [2]

a. **But are there effective COVID treatments?** Hundreds of studies done around the world have established, and repeatedly confirmed, **fast, effective, safe and well-tolerated treatments for COVID that are in widespread use**. I wrote about them in my book, *The Defeat of COVID: 500+ medical studies show what works & what doesn't.* [3]

To get started right away on reading the latest scientific information on early treatments for COVID, please see https://c19early.com. **All of the treatments in related webpages, such as https://c19ivermectin.com, https://c19hcq.com/ and https://vitamind.com have all shown far greater effectiveness and safety against COVID than any of the COVID vaccines.** That claim is bold, but it is overwhelmingly proven as indisputable fact in the hundreds of studies cited in this book.

b.   **General risk vs benefit**   An emergency experimental vaccine cannot be assumed to be safer than a virus with a very high survival rate, such as COVID. **The average survival rate for _NO_ COVID treatment at all is 99.85%, and we have very successful treatments available, which should easily achieve universal survivability from COVID, if widely available**. Where does 99.85% survival come from? Dr. John Ioannidis is one of the most widely cited scientists in the world. His estimate in June 2020 of a 0.26% infection fatality rate (IFR) had been confirmed around the world.   100% - 0.26% = 99.74% survival rate. That has now been revised to IFR = 0.15%. So 100% - 0.15% = 99.85% survival rate. [4]

2)   **Does the COVID vaccine work?** The COVID vaccine is not even known to stop the spread of COVID.

a.   Dr. Larry Corey, who oversees National Institutes of Health COVID vaccine trials said on 11/20/20: **_"The studies aren't designed to assess transmission. They don't ask that question, and there's really no information on this at this point in time."_** [5] Consider that this was right before the most widely deployed medical intervention of all time throughout the world. Was the public informed anywhere in the world that the vaccines were unknown to be able to stop spread of disease or infection? Since then, it has been seen that the earliest and most heavily vaccinated country, Israel, has had one of the highest COVID infection rates in the world since vaccination. [6]

b.   **The FDA confirmed back in December 2020 that the first vaccine dose correlates with increased COVID infections.**

"Suspected COVID cases that occurred within 7 days after any vaccination were 409 in the vaccine group vs 287 in the placebo group." This data comes from Pfizer itself. [7]

3)   **What happened to the animals in the studies?** This technology has been tried on animals, and in the animal studies done, *all the animals died following coronavirus vaccines*, not immediately, but months later, from other immune disorders, liver inflammation, [8] [9] and sepsis and/or cardiac failure. There has never been a long-term successful animal study using this technology. [10] No experimental coronavirus vaccine has succeeded in animal studies. [11]

4)   **Specific risks of COVID vaccines**, in roughly chronological order of side-effect manifestation:

a.   **Polyethylene glycol (PEG)** is one of the ingredients. This has been correlated with **anaphylactic shock.** [12] [13] **So the CDC began recommending intubation kits at vaccination sites**. [14]

b.   **Cationic lipid coating of mRNA** is known for many years to be toxic, [15] because these (+) charged fats interact with the (-) charges on our amino acids, our cell membranes and the phosphates of our DNA. Cationic lipids are attracted to and are destructive toward:

i.   Lungs [16]

ii.   Mitochondria, red blood cells, white blood cells [17]

iii.   Liver [18]

iv.   Nervous system (This is the Bell's Palsy and tremors that are seen in vaccine victims.) [19]

c.   **mRNA**: Unlike a traditional vaccine, of injected, inactivated virus intended to stimulate antibody response, the COVID vaccine on the other hand is completely different in this respect. It uses messenger RNA **(mRNA), which is a blueprint for your cells to create COVID-like (spike) proteins**. Then your cells begin to make these COVID-like proteins.

However, those proteins, in turn, stimulate your body to make antibodies against them. So now **your body has been turned into a munitions factory for both sides of a war**: The bad guys (COVID-like spike proteins) and the good guys (the antibodies fighting against them). However, before you pledge allegiance to the good guys, as you will see below, the good guys can be more lethal to the vaccinated person.

i.   **History of mRNA vaccines**: This technology had disastrous results in dengue fever vaccines in the past. Dengue vaccine is a mRNA vaccine. [20]

When this kind of technology, not identical to the mRNA COVID vaccines, but of a very narrowly targeted set of selected viral genes (from a different virus), was used in children in the Philippines, **many vaccinated children had far worse outcomes than unvaccinated children** when they were later exposed to dengue, and many died. Prosecution for homicide resulted. [21]   However, this had previously been known to happen with ferrets and with cats. In all cases, the vaccinated animal or human became *more* **vulnerable to worse disease** when confronted with it. It is expected that the relatively mild COVID illness, with a survival rate of 99.85%, may become more serious, with a much lower survival rate and become a truly lethal disease in vaccinated people when they later become infected with it. At this writing, (I wrote this chapter in February 2021) **there are no peer-reviewed published long-term human trials of mRNA vaccines at all**, and no mRNA vaccine has ever been FDA-approved. That's how new the technology is.

ii.   **mRNA can affect DNA**. One of the most worrisome risks with a mRNA vaccine is what can happen with reverse transcriptase. This is an enzyme in every cell, and it can theoretically lead to the **mRNA creating changes in the cells' DNA**, a process known as viral retro-integration.

Although this possibility had been thought unlikely, MIT and Harvard scientists found it happened here: [22]   If some of the 30 trillion or so cells in your body **become permanent COVID factories**, what is the long-term impact on your health, and would you want that outcome?

iii.   **Spike proteins cross the blood-brain barrier, attach to neurons and create brain inflammation**.   This is a problem because mRNA vaccines programmed the cells in the bodies of vaccinated people to keep making spike proteins. [23]

iv.   **Spike proteins directly damage lungs**. "*The researchers found that the genetically modified mice injected with the spike protein exhibited COVID-like symptoms that included severe inflammation, an influx of white blood cells into their lungs and evidence of a cytokine storm—an immune response in which the body starts to attack its own cells and tissues rather than just fighting off the virus. The mice that only received saline remained normal.*" [24]

v.   **Spike proteins likely damaged each of those organs due to: damage to mitochondria, which in turn damages vascular cells**, leading to the clotting and bleeding problems that we have now seen in COVID vaccine victims. "*S [spike] protein alone can damage endothelium.*" [25]

d.   **Antibody-dependent enhancement (ADE) problem:** Prior attempts to create a coronavirus vaccine killed all the test animals, after they were later infected with wild virus. Here's what happened: mRNA instructed the mammals' cells to produce the spike proteins of the coronavirus. Then, later, when the animals confronted the wild virus, **the intense build-up of antibodies had been stockpiled, and their sudden and overwhelming release killed the test animal**. These risks have been documented in *Nature*, *Science* and *Journal of Infectious Diseases*. Here's a study from the journal *Nature Microbiology* in September 2020 on that. [26]   Thus, long before even one person had received a COVID vaccine, this devastatingly poisonous effect was known by some and widely ignored.

e.   **ADE mechanism**: ADE is a form of pathogenic priming, meaning the vaccine can result in a more severe disease, which has been seen in prior attempts at making coronavirus vaccines. The antibodies made can be neutralizing (which inactivate a virus, and that's good).

However, antibodies are a problem when they are non-neutralizing, because then these antibodies carry active viruses directly to macrophages, which then become infected. This is how ADE happens.

This antibody dependent enhancement (ADE) leads to:

i.   increased viral replication (more viruses to make you sick); [27] and

ii.   more severe disease. [28]

f.   **ADE result**: These macrophages tend to go to the lungs and **fill the lungs, causing overwhelming inflammation and airway obstruction** (as found later on autopsy). [29]   However, the augmented antibodies also attack similar-looking proteins on internal organs, **resulting in cytokine storm and death,** [30] or **auto-immune disease and organ failure.** *"Cats that showed high titers following vaccination succumbed at later timepoints to fatal disease."* [31]

g.   **What about miscarriages, and why have men been advised to freeze their sperm prior to getting the injection?** Both men and women are at risk for possibly permanent infertility, because the spike protein of a coronavirus "looks" to the immune system similar to Syncytin-1, an essential protein in the placenta. This stimulates antibodies to fight the placenta, and possibly sperm. Mid-term miscarriages, which are normally very rare, have occurred in women who have been vaccinated for COVID. Miscarriages have increased by 3,016%. [32] [33] The New England Journal of Medicine had previously found that 14% of vaccinated pregnant women miscarried, mostly in the 3rd trimester, which is normally a very rare time to miscarry. [34]

Women should expect high risk of miscarriage and to remain infertile for an indefinite amount of time, possibly permanently, if they take the COVID vaccine. Also, SARS-CoV-2 viral particles have been found to linger in the testicles of men after recovery from infection. [35]

h.   **Myocarditis is a life-threatening condition**, which injures the muscular layer of the walls of the heart, **with no available treatment, because it entails the killing of heart cells**. Myocarditis is typically very rare in youth but has been disabling and killing vaccinated individuals. The CDC now confesses to the connection between myocarditis and the COVID vaccines. [36]

The following study shows the likely mechanism of harm done to the myocardium, [37] and everyone who takes the COVID vaccines would find it nearly impossible to reverse or prevent such permanent damage to the heart. I explain this mechanism. [38] [39]

Pathologist Roger Hodkinson MD explains the devastation of myocarditis:

> *"Myocarditis is never mild, particularly in young, healthy males. It's an inflammation of the heart muscle, the pump of the body. And we don't know what percent of the heart muscle cells would have died in any one attack of myocarditis. The big thing about heart muscle, heart muscle fibers, is that they do not regenerate . . . We do know that myocarditis can present decades later, with premature onset of heart failure that would otherwise not have been expected. So it's a terrible worry for these people to know what's going to happen to them in the future . . . It's not trivial"* [40]

i.   **Why are COVID vaccinees MORE likely to spread COVID than the unvaccinated?**

Virologist Geert Vanden Bossche PhD, who worked for the Bill & Melinda Gates Foundation, recently warned the World Health Organization (WHO) that "*We are currently turning vaccinees into carriers shedding infectious variants*."

The **Red Cross** says, "At this time individuals who have received a COVID vaccine are not able to donate convalescent plasma with the Red Cross." Pfizer showed awareness of the possibility of transmission through inhalation or skin contact with a vaccinated person here. See pages 67-68. [41] This may partly explain the spring-summer 2021 surge of anecdotal reports of unusual menstrual bleeding and clotting among contacts of vaccinated persons.

j.   **Why is it more dangerous to vaccinate against COVID than other viruses?** Because COVID virus uses the ACE-2 receptor to get into your endothelial cells, including those lining the blood vessels. This creates an inflammatory reaction that the great majority (99.85%) have survived (see above). So if you have been exposed to the virus, and then get vaccinated, it is almost certain that the vaccine will cause new inflammation and damage to endothelial cells lining your blood vessels, and we have seen abnormal blood clotting in people who have gotten the vaccine. But the more likely problem is launching new disease in the blood vessels. **Dr. H Noorchashm MD, PhD says, ". . . *the vaccine is almost certain to do damage to the vascular endothelium*.**" He explains in a letter that was deleted from its original sources, but may still be viewed. [42]

Israel is at this writing the most heavily COVID-vaccinated country in the world. The findings of infectious disease experts are reported here, [43] in which widely published infectious disease Professor Hervé Seligmann determined, from the Israeli data, that **the COVID vaccine causes:**

> "* . . .mortality hundreds of times greater in young people compared to mortality from coronavirus without the vaccine, and dozens of times more in the elderly . . .*"

---

5) **How to protect yourself and your family**

a. **As a physician, I strongly advise against this vaccine, regardless of brand, for everyone, without exception**.

b. **Always read the Product Package Insert**. This is required by law to be included with packaging of all vaccines, **and US Informed Consent Law protects your right to be fully informed prior to any medical procedure, and your right to reject any medical procedure**. 45 CFR § 46.116. [44] These are universal principles enshrined in the Nuremberg Code and the Universal Declaration of Human Rights, the Geneva Declaration of Medicine and the US Constitution.

Here is the Pfizer insert, [45] and here is Moderna's. [46] I strongly recommend reading ALL of it carefully with your family before you make a decision regarding whether to have the COVID vaccine.

c. Discuss the considerations above, as well as other information you have heard about the COVID vaccine in a relaxed, unhurried setting with your loved ones. **Make sure that you are not pressured** into a procedure that you may regret in the future. If you choose to defer or reject the COVID vaccine, know that you are not alone, and many healthcare workers have done the same. *"I've heard Tuskegee more times than I can count in the last month – and, you know, it's a valid, valid concern."* Dr. Nikhila Juvvadi, a hospital chief clinical officer. [47]

d. **Share this information sheet** with others who are also considering the vaccine.

e.   **If your employer or school attempts mandatory vaccination, show this information to them.** Federal law prohibits employers and others from requiring vaccination, such as the covid vaccine, that is under EUA (explained above). [48] You should also consult your attorney to look into state and federal law prohibiting forced medical procedures. Organizations such as the National Vaccine Information Center, [49] Children's Health Defense [50] and ICAN [51] may also have helpful information.

It is essential to avoid these vaccines by any legal means necessary. Dr. Peter McCullough, the most widely published cardiologist in human history, says:

> *"For the genetic vaccines, Pfizer, Moderna, Johnson and Johnson and Astra Zeneca, there is no known detoxification method. Sadly the genetic material lasts in the body far longer than what we thought, and the spike protein that's produced is probably in the body for greater than a year, and it's in vital areas, including the brain, the lung, the heart, the bone marrow, the reproductive organs. And it takes a very long time for the body to clear out this dangerous, foreign protein. The only thing I can advise individuals is, don't take any more of it. There is going to be a progressive accumulation of spike protein in the human body that cannot get out. It will almost certainly lead to chronic disease. Worldwide, the vaccine programs have backfired, meaning those countries that have the highest use of vaccines have the highest mortality rates."* [52]

f.   **If you find that the scientific information above is overwhelming, there is another way to look at COVID virus vs COVID vaccine risks.** How many famous people have died of COVID? How many famous people have died within 3 weeks after taking the COVID vaccine?

6)   **Fraud related to COVID vaccines**. The pharmaceutical industry is the largest advertiser in mainstream media. Journalists who lie* [53] about the COVID vaccines and masks are kept in their jobs. The above FDA finding of higher rates of COVID among the vaccinated than the unvaccinated has been confirmed by the FDA, and by Yale University public health professor and epidemiologist Harvey Risch. [54]

* (The journalist asked me for clarification; I provided her FDA webpage links with proof of the exact quote above, and *USA Today* published her false story regardless.)

The CDC announced a different COVID testing standard for unvaccinated people to deceptively multiply positive results by 4,096 times the positive COVID rate for unvaccinated people: https://www.cdc.gov/vaccines/COVID/downloads/Information-for-laboratories-COVID-vaccine-breakthrough-case-investigation.pdf, and then removed this document. There is also the egregiously deceptive propaganda that there is "a pandemic of the unvaccinated" based on the following sleight of hand: The CDC defines anyone as "unvaccinated" until more than two weeks after their 2nd COVID vaccine. [55] Therefore, acute injury, hospitalizations and deaths from the COVID vaccines are deceptively recorded as "unvaccinated."

Governments are pushing citizens intensely to take COVID vaccines, including with bribes, threats and/or coercion. Millions of people including healthcare workers are taking to the streets protesting these vaccine "mandates." Politicians and journalists must immediately stop trying to practice medicine. Their ignorance of basic immunology, microbiology and cardiology has led to reckless urging for people to take a poisonous injection, for which many people have lost their lives and others have sacrificed their health.

What we learned by 2022

Chapter 2

Court Testimony
on the COVID Vaccines:

The COVID Vaccines
Are Neither Safe Nor Effective

I have updated my January 2022 court testimony on deaths and hospitalizations correlated with the COVID vaccines, to incorporate recent data from governments in several countries.

The COVID vaccines are alarmingly and irredeemably unsafe, as well as ineffective for the advertised purposes. It is increasingly recognized by physicians, scientists and laypeople throughout the world that the COVID-19 vaccines are neither safe nor effective nor reversible, and I will provide the proof in this chapter.

Dr. Peter McCullough, cardiologist:

> *"For new biological products, we always demand, safety, safety, safety. . . . We have to discuss safety first. We always discuss safety, because if products are not safe, it doesn't matter how good they are. . . . Drugs don't go at all into commercial production if they are not safe."* [56]

Background

US mortality data at the end of 2020 did not support the allegation of a pandemic, because there was no more of an outlying peak in excess deaths in 2020 than other peaks throughout the past two decades. The CDC shows that 3,382,000 people died from all causes in the US in 2020, [57] remaining at about one percent of the total population, as in each of the previous three years, in which there was no pandemic. Notably, December 2020 had by far the highest deaths of any month in 2020 in the US, 32% higher than the average of the previous 11 months of what had been advertised to be the worst pandemic in a century, but in fact had no more than typical numbers of deaths in the US during that alleged pandemic.

It may be no coincidence that December 2020 was the month that the vaccines became available to the public. Early 2021 has shown striking excess deaths, and the COVID vaccine was the new factor, beginning the same week as excess deaths. Furthermore, January to November 2020 show an average of 274,000 deaths in the US per month, but since December 2020, according to the same CDC tables of data, the average deaths per month has jumped to 288,250. I will show in this paper that this increase in deaths in the US is most likely due to the new COVID vaccines that became available in December 2020, the same month that deaths in the US significantly increased.

The Pfizer COVID vaccines first became available for mass vaccination in the US on December 14, 2020, followed by the Moderna vaccine a few days later. The Johnson and Johnson vaccine would not become available till February 27, 2021. As soon as the earlier vaccines became distributed *en masse*, the total number of deaths per week for the rest of 2020 from all causes in the US jumped from 63,000 to 84,000, which is a 32% increase, unlikely to be attributable to any other cause but the vaccines.

It can be seen from the CDC data, that the deaths per week in the US in each of the first seven weeks following the Pfizer and Moderna rollout **_all_** exceeded even the deadliest weeks of 2020 (the two weeks ending April 11 and April 18 of 2020). [58] This should be enough to make anyone hesitant about the vaccines, and logically, more fearful of the vaccines than of COVID. In this chapter, I will share more published data and the latest scientific understanding of why the COVID vaccines are alarmingly and irredeemably unsafe, as well as ineffective for the advertised purpose of reducing COVID transmission, incidence, morbidity or mortality.

In BioNTech's (Pfizer's partner company) latest SEC filing, the company admitted to lack of proof of safety or efficacy of their vaccine -- in the same sentence -- in this PDF document: [59]

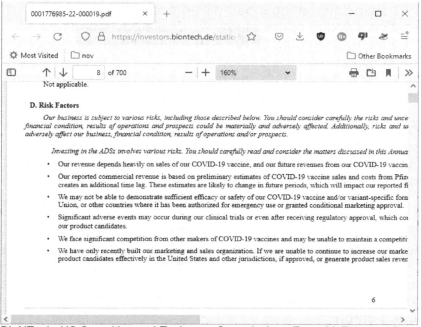

BioNTech. US Securities and Exchange Commission. Form 20-F Annual Report. Mar 30 2022. **https://investors.biontech.de/static-files/50d0cafc-b2c1-4392-a495-d252f84be105**

The COVID vaccines have negative efficacy, and what that means

The COVID vaccines are so ineffective against COVID that they have negative efficacy. I will explain what that is. Negative efficacy means that you have a greater likelihood of infection and / or hospitalization and / or deaths from COVID after having received the vaccine than not receiving it. The COVID vaccines have not only failed to reduce cases and hospitalizations from Omicron and COVID generally, but they have actually increased the incidence of both. Results of negative efficacy of the COVID vaccines are seen all over the world. Here is data to prove that:

Analysis of data from 145 countries shows that the COVID vaccines cause more COVID cases per million and more COVID-associated deaths per million over the vast international scope of this study. [60] The study found "a marked increase in both COVID-19 related cases and death due directly to a vaccine deployment . . . " The results in the US were 38% more cases per million [61] and 31% more deaths per million [62] caused by the COVID vaccines.

In order to comprehend this vast worldwide destructive effect of the COVID vaccines, let's now look at analyses of this phenomenon of negative efficacy of the vaccines in specific countries.

This Danish study [63] showed that both Pfizer and Moderna COVID vaccines showed negative efficacy against the Omicron variant within only 90 days of administration, and that that decline in efficacy is even faster for Omicron than for the Delta variant, which is no longer the predominant variant in the world at present. This sharp decline is illustrated in the following graph.

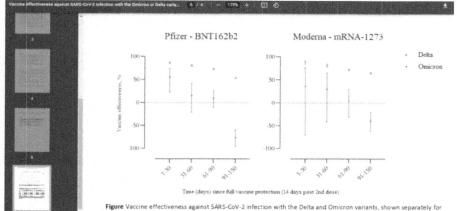

Figure Vaccine effectiveness against SARS-CoV-2 infection with the Delta and Omicron variants, shown separately for

C Hansen, A Schelde, et al. Vaccine effectiveness against SARS-CoV-2 infection with the Omicron or Delta variants following a two-dose or booster BNT162b2 or mRNA-1273 vaccination series: A Danish cohort study.
https://www.medrxiv.org/content/10.1101/2021.12.20.21267966v3.full.pdf

The above graph shows that both of the mRNA COVID vaccines predispose toward increased risk, due to negative efficacy, for Omicron especially and to a lesser extent, Delta, which at this writing is a variant no longer in circulation.

89.7% of people infected with Omicron in Denmark are either "fully vaccinated" or had their first booster. 77.9% of the Danish population is fully vaccinated. [64] Therefore, the vaccinated have been more predisposed to Omicron infection than the unvaccinated in Denmark.

Data from the United Kingdom (UK) government, Office for National Statistics, shows that each successive vaccine dose has increased the likelihood of testing positive for the Omicron variant, in a stunning display of negative vaccine efficacy, as seen in the tables below. [65]

Table 1b

Modelled likelihood of testing positive with an Omicron probable result in people who test positive for COVID-19, by screened dem
29 November 2021 to 12 December 2021

Screening characteristic	Category	Estimated likelihood of testing positive for COVID-19 with an Omicron probable result (odds ratio)	Lower 95% confidence interval	Upper 95% confidence interval	p-value
Vaccination status	Not vaccinated (*Reference*)	1	-	-	-
Vaccination status	1 dose	1.57	0.52	4.54	0.413
Vaccination status	2 doses, more than 14 days ago	2.26	0.78	7.45	0.157
Vaccination status	3 doses, more than 14 days ago	4.45	1.29	17.03	0.023
Previous COVID-19 infection	No (*Reference*)	1	-	-	-
Previous COVID-19 infection	Yes	3.22	1.31	7.29	0.007
Work Status	Employed, working (*Reference)*	1	-	-	-
Work Status	Employed, not working	0.67	0.08	4.20	0.725
Work Status	Not working	0.70	0.19	1.97	0.537
Work Status	Retired	0.94	0.28	3.02	0.919
Work Status	Child/student	1.62	0.41	6.39	0.486
Travel abroad status (in the last 28 days)	No (Reference)	1	-	-	-
Travel abroad status (in the last 28 days)	Yes	4.60	2.41	8.62	0.000

Source: Office for National Statistics - Coronavirus (COVID-19) Infection Survey

Worse yet, risk of death from COVID-19 is shown to increase with each successive dose of vaccine for most age groups, as in the following table published by the UK government's Health Security Agency. [66]

COVID-19 vaccine surveillance report – week 9

Table 12. COVID-19 deaths (a) within 28 days and (b) within 60 days of positive specimen or with COVID-19 reported on death certificate, by vaccination status between week 5 2022 and week 8 2022
Please note that corresponding rates by vaccination status can be found in Table 13.
(a)

Death within 28 days of positive COVID-19 test by date of death between week 5 2022 (w/e 6 February 2022) and week 8 2022 (w/e 27 February 2022)	Total**	Unlinked*	Not vaccinated	Received one dose (1 to 20 days before specimen date)	Received one dose, ≥21 days before specimen date	Second dose ≥14 days before specimen date[1]	Third dose ≥14 days before specimen date[1]
			[This data should be interpreted with caution. See information below in footnote about the correct interpretation of these figures]				
Under 18	4	0	3	0	1	0	0
18 to 29	10	0	3	0	1	4	2
30 to 39	27	1	11	0	1	8	6
40 to 49	73	2	21	1	6	24	19
50 to 59	172	3	45	1	15	43	65
60 to 69	353	3	48	0	15	78	209
70 to 79	827	5	96	0	22	155	549
80 or over	2,491	4	170	0	50	413	1,854

* Individuals whose NHS numbers were unavailable to link to the NIMS.
** number of deaths of people who had had a positive test result for COVID-19 and either died within 60 days of the first positive test or have COVID-19 mentioned on their death certificate.
[1] In the context of very high vaccine coverage in the population, even with a highly effective vaccine, it is expected that a large proportion of cases, hospitalisations and deaths would occur in vaccinated individuals, simply because a larger proportion of the population are vaccinated than unvaccinated and no vaccine is 100% effective. This is especially true because vaccination has been prioritised in individuals who are more susceptible or more at risk of severe disease. Individuals in risk groups may also be more at risk of hospitalisation or death due to non-COVID-19 causes, and thus may be hospitalised or die with COVID-19 rather than because of COVID-19.

For UK children, the vaccines are especially deadly. The UK Office for Statistics reports that British children are up to 52 times more likely to die following a COVID vaccine. The damage was shown to be dose-dependent. For children aged 15 to 19, the risk of death nearly doubles if they take the first injection and becomes triple if they receive the second injection. [67] [68] The reader may verify this by dividing the number of all deaths by person-years per dose and for each age group. (GOV.UK no longer shows Table 9 -May 2022.)

Table 9: Whole period counts of deaths and person-years by vaccination status and five year age group, England, deaths occurring between 1 January 2021 and 31 October 2021

Vaccination status	Age group	Person-years	Deaths involving COVID-19	Non-COVID-19 deaths	All deaths
Received only the first dose, at least 21 days ago	10-14	6,648	0	3	3
Received only the first dose, at least 21 days ago	15-19	176,667	0	32	32

Table 9, ONS Report

Table 9: Whole period counts of deaths and person-years by vaccination status and five year age group, England, deaths occurring between 1 January 2021 and 31 October 2021[1]

Vaccination status	Age group	Person-years	Deaths involving COVID-19	Non-COVID-19 deaths	All deaths
Received the second dose, at least 21 days ago	10-14	1,678	0	4	4
Received the second dose, at least 21 days ago	15-19	127,842	1	41	42

Table 9, ONS Report

Table 9: Whole period counts of deaths and person-years by vaccination status and five year age group, England, deaths occurring between 1 January 2021 and 31 October 2021[1]

Vaccination status	Age group	Person-years	Deaths involving COVID-19	Non-COVID-19 deaths	All deaths
Unvaccinated	10-14	2,094,711	2	94	96
Unvaccinated	15-19	1,587,072	18	142	160

Table 9, ONS Report

See Endnote 67 for source and more readable, author-re-typed version of table.

Astonishingly, as bad as this threat is for older teens, it was even worse for younger teens. Whereas there were 32.9 deaths per 100,000 person-years among 15 to 19 year olds, there were 238.4 deaths per 100,000 person-years among 10 to 14 year-olds in the UK. These data may be calculated from the above tables.

On a population wide level in Ireland, mass vaccination is correlated in timing with dramatically rising COVID-19 cases.

The Irish population has among the highest rates of vaccine penetration in its adult population, 94.8% fully vaccinated as of January 22, 2022, yet COVID-19 cases rose 317% over the previous January, before the vaccines were in use. [69]

In Scotland also, among those who had received one, two or three vaccines, or none at all, the unvaccinated had the lowest case rates in January 2022 of all four groups, as seen in this graph. [70]

Figure 13: COVID-19 age-standardised case rate per 100,000 individuals by vaccine status, seven-day rolling average from 10 May 2021 to 14 January 2022.

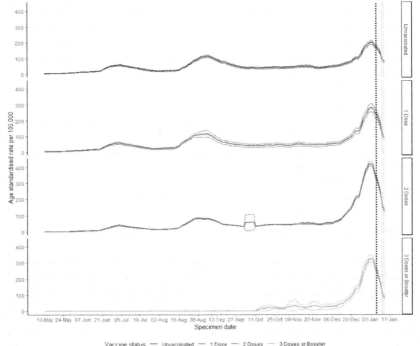

Public Health Scotland. Public Health Scotland COVID-19 & Winter Statistical Report. Jan 17 2022. **https://publichealthscotland.scot/media/11802/22-01-19-covid19-winter_publication_report_revised.pdf**

Scotland has also shown record-breaking rates of newborn deaths since the advent of COVID vaccination. [71]   Many vaccinations of pregnant mothers happened before Pfizer was forced to disclose their mortality and morbidity figures by court order. Here are those infant deaths.

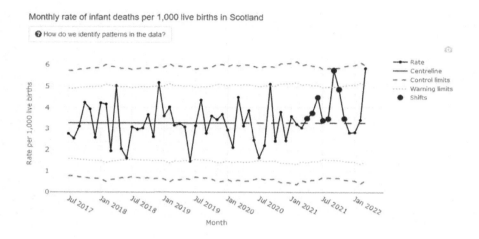

Monthly rate of infant deaths per 1,000 live births in Scotland

Two other very heavily vaccinated countries have seen their case rates skyrocket since mass vaccination. Following are Germany and South Korea COVID-19 cases per million people. [72]

Daily new confirmed COVID-19 cases per million people

7-day rolling average. Due to limited testing, the number of confirmed cases is lower than the true number of infections.

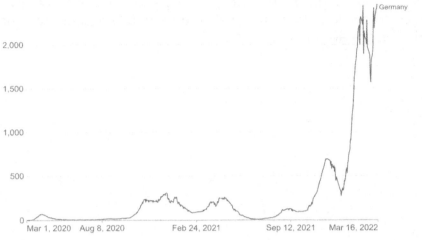

Source: Johns Hopkins University CSSE COVID-19 Data

CC BY

Daily new confirmed COVID-19 cases per million people

7-day rolling average. Due to limited testing, the number of confirmed cases is lower than the true number of infections.

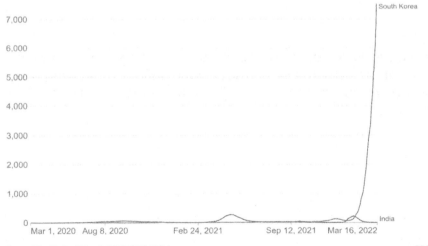

Source: Johns Hopkins University CSSE COVID-19 Data

CC BY

Johns Hopkins University. Our World in Data.
https://ourworldindata.org/coronavirus#explore-the-global-situation

Lack of efficacy of the COVID vaccines is seen in Germany. The German data show that from the 4,020 cases of Omicron in Germany on December 31, 2021. Of those, 1,137 were boosted. Of note, there were only 1097 unvaccinated Omicron cases. [73] [74] [75] However, there were similar numbers of people in the three categories of "boosted," fully vaccinated" and "unvaccinated" in Germany as of 12/31/21. German scientists studying the German government's excess mortality data observed that the higher the vaccination rate, the higher the excess mortality. [76]

As we can see, the unvaccinated have had a strong advantage against Omicron, which was the prevalent COVID strain throughout the world at that time. The COVID vaccines do not work against the Delta strain either. In July 2021, in the United States, in Massachusetts, at a time and place that Delta was predominant, of a total of 469 new COVID cases, 346 of those (74%) were in people who were partially or fully vaccinated, and 274 of the vaccinated were symptomatic. [77]

In Delhi, India, of 34 Omicron cases at a hospital, 33 were fully vaccinated (97%). However, India's COVID vaccination rate was only 40% at that time. [78]

In Canada, during the week of April 10 to 17, 2022, 99.6% of deaths diagnosed as COVID deaths were in vaccinated people. [79] [80] In contrast, 84.83% of Canada's population is vaccinated with at least one dose. [81] These data are all from the Canadian government official sites.

The COVID vaccines have had disastrous results in Israel as well. Mass vaccination began in Israel on December 19, 2020. Nearly every Israeli adult has received two or more doses of the Pfizer vaccine. Since then, death spikes have reached much higher than previously over the last two years. This graph is from Johns Hopkins University statistics.

In the following graph, December 19, 2020 is marked, because that is when mass vaccination began in Israel.

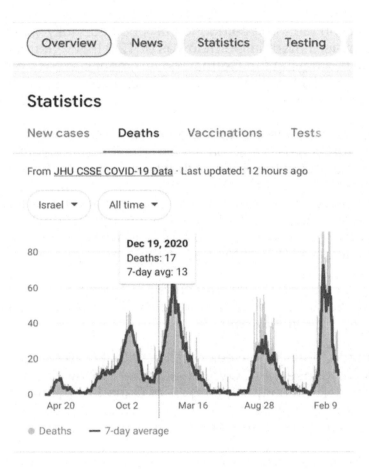

If the COVID vaccines merely predisposed one to higher risk of the common cold now known as the Omicron and Delta variants, then we might simply laugh off these vaccines as a frivolous and superstitious activity. However, the safety data are nothing less than horrifying, as will be seen in the next section of this chapter.

There is an additional problem implied by the COVID vaccines' negative efficacy. That is, that the fully vaccinated have been experiencing Antibody Dependent Enhancement and VAIDS or vaccine-acquired immune-deficiency syndrome. This means that, according to consistent evidence from around the world, the immune systems of vaccinated people have been weakened to the point where they cannot fight a SARS-CoV-2 infection as well as unvaccinated people, most likely due to the mechanisms that I discuss in the Chapter 1 of this book.

As of this time, no children have died in the United States with a COVID diagnosis except for those having terminal leukemia and other advanced cancers and grave terminal illnesses. It has been calculated that seasonal flu, lightning and being a passenger in a motor vehicle are all more life-threatening to children and adolescents than any of the COVID variants.

The COVID vaccines are not safe

The decision to vaccinate and its impacts are irreversible. There is now considerable evidence of harm and deaths caused by the COVID vaccines. The COVID vaccines are known to be hazardous, because of the 1,223 deaths acknowledged by Pfizer and the FDA, as shown below in this screenshot from Pfizer's documentation, released only under court order, the same documentation that the FDA sought to have sealed for 55 years, and then for 75 years, but was forced to be released under court order. Pfizer's document is now accessible to the public, including the table below. [82]

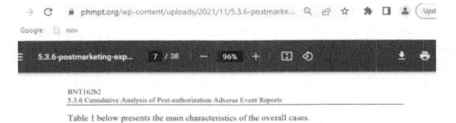

BNT162b2
5.3.6 Cumulative Analysis of Post-authorization Adverse Event Reports

Table 1 below presents the main characteristics of the overall cases.

Table 1. General Overview: Selected Characteristics of All Cases Received During the Reporting Interval

Characteristics		Relevant cases (N=42086)
Gender:	Female	29914
	Male	9182
	No Data	2990
Age range (years):	≤ 17	175ª
0.01 -107 years	18-30	4953
Mean = 50.9 years	31-50	13886
n = 34952	51-64	7884
	65-74	3098
	≥ 75	5214
	Unknown	6876
Case outcome:	Recovered/Recovering	19582
	Recovered with sequelae	520
	Not recovered at the time of report	11361
	Fatal	1223
	Unknown	9400

a. in 46 cases reported age was <16-year-old and in 34 cases <12-year-old.

Aside from the 1223 deaths, please notice the preceding line in the above table: the 11,361 cases "not recovered at the time of report."

Pfizer also confessed over 1,500 types of adverse reactions, many of them known to be permanently disabling, as documented in court-ordered FDA document release on the adverse events observed after administration of the Pfizer vaccine in the clinical trials. [83] [84] [85] The clinical trials of the Pfizer vaccine showed tremendously concerning data, which was not initially shared with the general public, and has had to be extracted by court order and numerous FOIA requests. This document summarizes the problems with the trial, and the vaccine hazards that became apparent from the trial. [86]

The Vaccine Adverse Events Reporting Service (VAERS) was established by the US Department of Health and Human Services (HHS) to track vaccine related injuries and deaths. It is the only central database for vaccine injuries and deaths in the US for healthcare providers to record such events. More deaths and injuries have now been reported on VAERS following the COVID vaccines in just one year of use than for all other vaccines **_combined_** over the last 30 years of reporting, at this writing numbering over 27,000 deaths in the US alone from the COVID vaccines. [87] [88]

New drugs are generally pulled immediately from the market in the US, per FDA standards, after 50 deaths. But the COVID vaccines for some reason have had protection against evidence of human suffering and death. Over 50,000 Americans are now permanently disabled following deployment of these vaccines. [89] [90]

Data analysis of incidence of stroke in the same VAERS system of the US Dept of Health and Human Services shows the following: From December 2020 to February 11 2022, 4,532 adverse events following vaccination involved a stroke. That was a 14-month period. However, there were only 122 adverse events following flu shots from 2008 to 2020. That was a 13-year period. So the COVID vaccines are considerably riskier than the flu shots for stroke alone.

Per dose administered, the VAERS data shows that stroke is over 11,000% more likely to happen after a COVID vaccine than a flu shot. [91] [92]

But the comparison gets worse. The following chart shows a comparison, derived from data in VAERS, of the number of flu shots given for each death vs the number of COVID-19 vaccines given per each death. [93] [94]

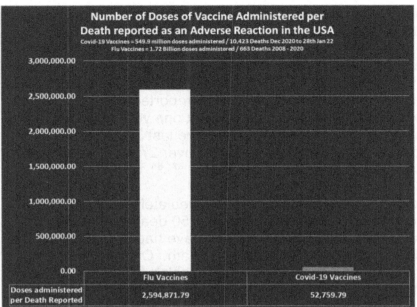

The Exposé. FACT: Covid-19 vaccines are almost 50 times deadlier than the flu vaccines per number of doses administered according to official USA data. Feb 21 2022. **https://dailyexpose.uk/2022/02/21/covid-vaccines-50-times-deadlier-than-flu-vaccines/**.

We can see that the COVID-19 vaccines are 49 times deadlier than the flu vaccines. (This author has treated many times over the years patients who were permanently disabled following a flu shot, and the COVID vaccines are shown by US government data to be 49 times as deadly.)

Pfizer data released by the FDA upon court order showed reports of 1,223 deaths among vaccinated people within the first 90 days following vaccine administration. [95] The FDA, on behalf of Pfizer, had requested 75 years to release 450,000 pages of data, but this was denied by a federal judge. [96] And fraud has been verified in the Pfizer vaccine trial, including falsifying data, unblinding patients, being slow to follow up on adverse events, mis-labelled laboratory specimens, and the targeting and firing of staff for reporting these types of problems. [97]

On the next page is a screenshot of just part of the first page (alphabetically) of adverse events that the FDA and Pfizer admitted to the Court under Court order, not even including all that begin with the letter A. [98]

I apologize in advance to the reader for mentioning at least five times throughout this book the above data confessed by Pfizer and the FDA only under court order regarding the 1,223 deaths, over 1,500 different types of health effects and over 158,000 distinct individual injuries found during the clinical trials. If one were writing about the Nazi Holocaust, one might mention more than once all the six million Jews who were killed in that particular blight on human history.

The newer holocaust that is now unfolding, insidiously peaceful in its appearance, and slow in its effects, is a worldwide event, and it is essential to remember that court-order revealed data were absolutely cautionary, even prohibitive, to the use of COVID vaccines in any humans, except with un-coerced and informed consent in voluntary human clinical trials, and even then, only after successful animal trials. Certainly, tyrannical measures to force vaccination on people could never be justified in a post-Nuremberg world.

Would anyone who had access to this information before being vaccinated have consented to receive these vaccines?

Let's look at what Pfizer knew and confessed to the Court on the following page.

BNT162b2
5.3.6 Cumulative Analysis of Post-authorization Adverse Event Reports

APPENDIX 1. LIST OF ADVERSE EVENTS OF SPECIAL INTEREST

1p36 deletion syndrome;2-Hydroxyglutaric aciduria;5'nucleotidase increased;Acoustic neuritis;Acquired C1 inhibitor deficiency;Acquired epidermolysis bullosa;Acquired epileptic aphasia;Acute cutaneous lupus erythematosus;Acute disseminated encephalomyelitis;Acute encephalitis with refractory, repetitive partial seizures;Acute febrile neutrophilic dermatosis;Acute flaccid myelitis;Acute haemorrhagic leukoencephalitis;Acute haemorrhagic oedema of infancy;Acute kidney injury;Acute macular outer retinopathy;Acute motor axonal neuropathy;Acute motor-sensory axonal neuropathy;Acute myocardial infarction;Acute respiratory distress syndrome;Acute respiratory failure;Addison's disease;Administration site thrombosis;Administration site vasculitis;Adrenal thrombosis;Adverse event following immunisation;Ageusia;Agranulocytosis;Air embolism;Alanine aminotransferase abnormal;Alanine aminotransferase increased;Alcoholic seizure;Allergic bronchopulmonary mycosis;Allergic oedema;Alloimmune hepatitis;Alopecia areata;Alpers disease;Alveolar proteinosis;Ammonia abnormal;Ammonia increased;Amniotic cavity infection;Amygdalohippocampectomy;Amyloid arthropathy;Amyloidosis;Amyloidosis senile;Anaphylactic reaction;Anaphylactic shock;Anaphylactic transfusion reaction;Anaphylactoid reaction;Anaphylactoid shock;Anaphylactoid syndrome of pregnancy;Angioedema;Angiopathic neuropathy;Ankylosing spondylitis;Anosmia;Antiacetylcholine receptor antibody positive;Anti-actin antibody positive;Anti-aquaporin-4 antibody positive;Anti-basal ganglia antibody positive;Anti-cyclic citrullinated peptide antibody positive;Anti-epithelial antibody positive;Anti-erythrocyte antibody positive;Anti-exosome complex antibody positive;Anti-GAD antibody negative;Anti-GAD antibody positive;Anti-ganglioside antibody positive;Antigliadin antibody positive;Anti-glomerular basement membrane antibody positive;Anti-glomerular basement membrane disease;Anti-glycyl-tRNA synthetase antibody positive;Anti-HLA antibody test positive;Anti-IA2 antibody positive;Anti-insulin antibody increased;Anti-insulin antibody positive;Anti-insulin receptor antibody increased;Anti-insulin receptor antibody positive;Anti-interferon antibody negative;Anti-interferon antibody positive;Anti-islet cell antibody positive;Antimitochondrial antibody positive;Anti-muscle

Again, this is only the first part of the letter A in Pfizer's alphabetical list of the carnage suffered with these vaccines. The reader is urged to read the entire list here. [99]

The US military has experienced an 1100% increase in deaths in one of the youngest and fittest cohorts in the US population, the military's own recruits, as revealed in US Senate testimony.

Data from the military's DMED system show that cancer diagnoses tripled in recruits after the deployment of the COVID vaccines, and that this primarily comprises a young population. That data may only be submitted to the DMED system by military doctors [100]

Because of the deaths and injuries witnessed as a result of the COVID vaccines as well as violation of civil liberties and human rights, the US Navy Seals are prosecuting the Biden Administration. [101]

Independent data analysts have determined, using nine different types of analysis, that the number of Americans that have been killed by the COVID vaccines now likely numbers approximately 388,000, but is at least 150,000. [102] [103] This number is consistent with the increase in weekly deaths reported by the CDC in the first seven weeks of vaccine availability. There was an average of 84,896 all-cause deaths in the US per week in those first horrific seven weeks of vaccine rollout, as referenced in the first page of this report. Whereas there were only 63,340 all-cause deaths in the US per week throughout 2020 (during allegedly the worst pandemic in a century) prior to vaccine rollout, there was an average of 84,896 deaths during those seven weeks post-rollout. This is an estimated excess of 150,885 Americans who died during those seven weeks beginning with the Pfizer rollout. For perspective, the swine flu vaccine was pulled off the US market in 1976 after only 25 deaths.

The peer-reviewed medical literature is replete with studies showing injuries and deaths correlated to the COVID vaccines. Here are over 1,000 such studies and reports on PubMed, which is the largest medical library in the world. [104] Among these studies there are 90 studies on myocarditis and acute myocarditis alone following the COVID vaccines.

Individual doctors also report significant increases in morbidity. Rheumatologist Robert Jackson MD has practiced medicine for 35 years. Of his approximately 5,000 patients, approximately 3,000 were vaccinated with the COVID vaccines. 40% of those patients reported a vaccine injury. Although he would typically see one or two deaths per year among his patients, there have been 12 deaths in the past year among the vaccinated. [105] Dr. Jackson's findings are comparable to those in the published medical literature, and in the 30-country EULAR study. [106]

Mechanisms by which the COVID vaccines cause injury

World renowned microbiologist Sucharit Bhakdi shows that 93% of people who died after the COVID vaccine were killed by the vaccine, and that the pathology of those autopsied showed life-threatening effects throughout the body. [107]

The preponderance of evidence so far is that the principal mechanism of damage to various bodily organs is by means of micro-clotting, due to disruption of normally smooth, laminar, unimpeded liquid blood flow through the circulatory system, now cluttered with jutting spike proteins from the endothelium into the lumen of capillaries, where a now overburdened heart must push – no longer smooth liquid blood – but now turbulent, and then micro-clotted and somewhat jellied blood through where liquid blood used to flow easily, freely and without obstruction. [108] [109] [110]

It has now been found that two-thirds of adolescents with COVID vaccine-related myopericarditis sustained continued heart abnormalities for months after their initial diagnosis. This has been verified with late gadolinium enhancement (LGE) on cardiac MRI imaging. Such findings are in alignment with the well-established cardiology observation and understanding that neither myocarditis nor myopericarditis is an acute or transitory condition, but rather these serious diseases involve death of irreplaceable cardiomyocytes, which are necessary for the health and proper function of heart muscle and the heart's ability to pump blood. [111]

The Pfizer COVID vaccines have also been observed to damage the human innate immune system, [112] and specifically an aspect of our immunity that is necessary to fight viral infections, and to result in "weak T-cell responses," and to even interfere with immune system responses to other vaccinations. [113]

The UK government acknowledges what mRNA technology scientists have known for decades: The COVID vaccines are a form of gene therapy, which rely on lipid carriers. [114]

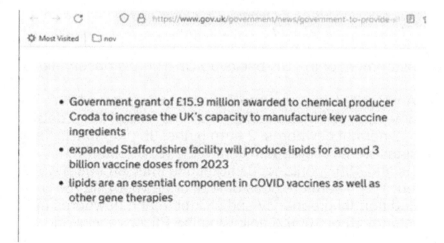

- Government grant of £15.9 million awarded to chemical producer Croda to increase the UK's capacity to manufacture key vaccine ingredients
- expanded Staffordshire facility will produce lipids for around 3 billion vaccine doses from 2023
- lipids are an essential component in COVID vaccines as well as other gene therapies

This was also confessed by BioNTech, Pfizer's COVID vaccine partner, in their Mar 30 2021 SEC Annual Report filing. [115]

In lipid envelopes, the mRNA in COVID vaccines can be transported across the blood-brain barrier. Now psychosis and other psychiatric pathologies are being observed following the COVID vaccines. This is correlated with altered findings on brain imaging. [116]

In summary, I agree with the World Health Organization Director General Tedros Adhanom Ghebreyesus that boosters should not be used to kill children.[117] Why would he suggest that the vaccines are being used to kill children, when enthusiastic adults want to give the COVID vaccines to their children?

Dr. James Thorp, a 68-year-old obstetrician/gynecologist, has practiced obstetrics for 42 years. He sees 6,000 to 7,000 high risk pregnancies per year, and Dr. Thorp says:

> *"What I've seen in the last two years is unprecedented: many, many, many complications due to the COVID vaccines, in pregnant women, in moms and in fetuses, in children . . . fetal death, miscarriage . . . unprecedented."* [118]

The Government of the UK backs up Dr. Thorp's observations:

In the April 2022 Pfizer vaccine data compiled by the UK Government, possibly exclusively from the Yellow Card data system, 2 normal newborns, 2 term births, 35 pregnancies and 8 live births were recorded. In contrast 2 fetal deaths 10 stillbirths and 489 spontaneous abortions (miscarriages) were recorded. [119] Therefore, loss of fetal or newborn life (501) exceeded normal pregnancy and childbirth and newborns (47) by a factor of 10 or 1066%, following the Pfizer vaccine in pregnant women.

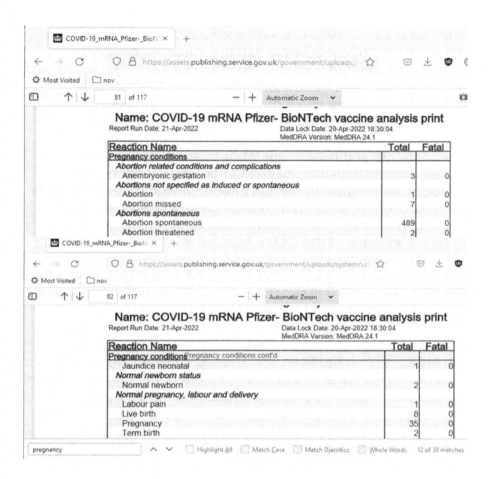

Name: COVID-19 mRNA Pfizer- BioNTech vaccine analysis print

Report Run Date: 21-Apr-2022   Data Lock Date: 20-Apr-2022 18:30:04
MedDRA Version: MedDRA 24.1

Reaction Name	Total	Fatal
Pregnancy conditions		
Abortion related conditions and complications		
Anembryonic gestation	3	0
Abortions not specified as induced or spontaneous		
Abortion	1	0
Abortion missed	7	0
Abortions spontaneous		
Abortion spontaneous	489	0
Abortion threatened	2	0

Name: COVID-19 mRNA Pfizer- BioNTech vaccine analysis print

Report Run Date: 21-Apr-2022   Data Lock Date: 20-Apr-2022 18:30:04
MedDRA Version: MedDRA 24.1

Reaction Name	Total	Fatal
Pregnancy conditions Pregnancy conditions cont'd		
Jaundice neonatal	1	0
Normal newborn status		
Normal newborn	2	0
Normal pregnancy, labour and delivery		
Labour pain	1	0
Live birth	8	0
Pregnancy	35	0
Term birth	2	0

pregnancy   ∧ ∨   ☐ Highlight All ☐ Match Case ☐ Match Diacritics ☐ Whole Words   12 of 38 matches

The Canadian COVID Care Alliance:

> "Recent studies [120] [121] [122] suggest that the spike protein produced in response to vaccination, may bind and interact with various cells throughout the body, via their ACE2 receptors, potentially resulting in damage to various tissues and organs. This risk, no matter how theoretical, must be investigated prior to the vaccination of children and adolescents."

The Canadian COVID Care Alliance calls on the Canadian government "to Immediately halt the mass vaccination program of children and adolescents until such time as studies are conducted and the uncertainties about the potential pathogenicity of the spike protein can be addressed." Here is their letter, signed by 21 scientists, to Ontario Premier Ford regarding the same. [123] I agree with this, and I urge governments and healthcare leaders and providers and independently thinking citizens to take the precautionary principle with regard to human health. It would be reckless to vaccinate either children or adults, given the abundant and growing evidence that we have seen of the dangers and negative efficacy of the COVID vaccines.

It is important to keep in mind that those of us who have been warning about the lethal nature of the COVID vaccines – and I have been warning the public against them since February 2021 [124] – expect that these vaccines cause slow cumulative damage to especially the heart, [125] [126] the immune system, [127] the brain, [128] and the liver. [129] The COVID vaccines are highly concerning for subsequent development of cancer, because of the abundant spike proteins produced by the vaccines, and their observed role in inhibiting DNA damage repair. [130] They are also concerning for female fertility, because of the high concentration found in the ovaries. [131] [132] This means that although the COVID vaccines have already been disastrous in terms of lives lost, the larger vaccine catastrophe is likely yet to arrive, even if no more injections are given.

Chapter 3

Bradford Hill criteria applied to COVID vaccines

Do the COVID vaccines meet the Bradford Hill criteria for causation of injuries and deaths?

How do we know if society-wide changes are responsible for health effects in populations? Population-wide environmental factors may or may not be related to subsequent health changes in the population and present difficulty in determining cause and effect, especially if multiple large-scale events happen in a close time frame.

Sir Austin Bradford Hill published a set of criteria to assess for or to determine epidemiological causality in 1965.   [133] These have become generally accepted standards for assessing which causes can be reasonably tied to which effects in our infinitely variable, often chaotic and abundantly populated world.

Let's consider the example of the city of Flint, Michigan, which in early 2015 experienced a rise in lead content of its municipal tap water from 104 parts per billion (ppb) to a 707 ppb in only two months, and in some places over 13,000 ppb. [134] [135]   To put that in perspective, the Environmental Protection Agency (EPA) established an upper safety limit of 15 ppb in drinking water.

As might be expected, Flint residents soon showed widespread clinical signs and symptoms that were consistent with known effects of lead poisoning, such as skin rashes, nausea, hair loss and anxiety and depression. [136] Such signs and symptoms of lead toxicity had been known for centuries, and are well-documented by toxicologists. But were these caused by lead in their water, or by something else? There were other data that met Bradford Hill criteria, which led to the conclusion of cause and effect between the higher than usual levels of lead found in Flint drinking water and observed signs and symptoms of poisoning in the Flint population.

A half-century later after Bradford Hill published his list, causality criteria were in place to assess if the clinical presentations of Flint residents were likely related to the sudden spike of lead contamination in their drinking water, as opposed to other possible mass-scale causes.

Hill's criteria can be summarized as follows:

1) <u>Strength of Association</u>: Are there very different findings among populations with different environmental exposures? Is one population much more likely to experience a common effect than another, in which the two populations differ in some environmental exposure? If so, by what factor or rate of prevalence of an observed health parameter?

2) <u>Consistency</u>: Do independent observers see the same pattern or association between two variables being considered? Is the association observed among multiple populations, or across multiple studies by different authors? If there are animal studies, are the findings in humans consistent with the findings in the animal studies?

3) <u>Specificity</u>: Does the substance of exposure cause a specific set of diseases or symptoms?

4) <u>Temporality</u>: Does exposure precede the onset of a disease or condition? How close in time?

5) <u>Biological gradient, or dose-response</u>: Does greater exposure correlate with more incidence of disease or more severe clinical effects?

6) <u>Plausibility</u>: Does a cause-effect relationship between the two variables make sense from a point of view of a commonly held understanding of biochemistry or physiology and known toxicology data?

7) <u>Coherence</u>: Does everything about the cause-effect possibility make sense, and stand the test of time and different ways of analyzing the data?

8) <u>Experiment</u>: Does greater exposure produce more effect? Does discontinuance of exposure reduce or eliminate the effect?

9) <u>Analogy</u>: Does a similar agent cause a similar disease?

Since the international release of the COVID vaccines in December 2020, there have been anomalous health events reported around the world. But is there a cause-and-effect relationship between the vaccines and human health events, including higher rates of deaths from all causes, cardiovascular injury and COVID positivity? Some of the following analysis refers to and relies on data reported in Chapter 2 of this book, [137] and a reader of that chapter will find a few of the references below familiar, but there are also newer data that I cite below.

A wide variety of human health events, that differed in incidence and prevalence from before, has been reported following administration of the COVID vaccines. Let's apply Bradford Hill's nine criteria one at a time, as follows, in order to see if a causal relationship between the COVID vaccines on the one hand, and increased injuries, infections and deaths on the other hand, is likely or not.

1) **Strength of association** may be seen in vaccinated versus unvaccinated populations. We can see there is a difference expressed in the government health statistics of a number of countries.

Our World In Data (**https://ourworldindata.org/**) is the largest public health database at this time in the world. It is cited by *Nature*, *Science*, *The New York Times*, *The Washington Post* and *The Wall Street Journal*. It is used in teaching at Harvard, Stanford, Berkeley and Oxford.

Analysis of that worldwide data shows that the higher the rate of vaccination in a country, the higher the COVID death rate. Data analyst Joel Smalley shows from these data that the greater percentage of vaccination of a country's population, the higher the COVID mortality rate, along the blue line in the graph below. Each dot represents a country. [138]

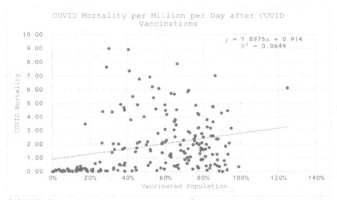

J Smalley. COVID Requiem Aeternam. https://metatron.substack.com/p/covid-requiem-aeternam

Smalley's summary of the 202 countries studied shows the following:

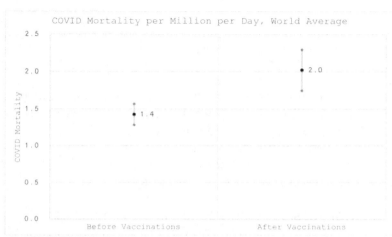

J Smalley. COVID Requiem Aeternam.
https://metatron.substack.com/p/covid-requiem-aeternam

Pfizer data showed that the vaccinated cohort had different rates of certain types of injuries than the unvaccinated. There were over 1,223 deaths and 158,000 adverse events among vaccinated people observed in the Pfizer clinical trials within the first 90 days after vaccine administration, [139] and this information was released by Pfizer and the FDA only under court order. [140]

From CDC data, the association of COVID vaccine uptake with death is 49 times stronger than the flu shot in the US. [141] Although the vaccines have only been available for about 16 months at this writing, already over 27,000 Americans have died, and over 50,000 Americans are permanently disabled after one or more doses of these vaccines. [142] [143]

Official data from the US Centers for Disease Control and Prevention (CDC) [144] [145] show that 12,548 children had serious adverse events, and 106 children died following COVID vaccines as of April 22, 2022.

Age	Events Reported	Percent (of 12,548)
< 6 months	61	0.49%
6-11 months	19	0.15%
1-2 years	32	0.26%
3-5 years	347	2.77%
6-17 years	12,089	96.34%
Total	12,548	100.00%

The Exposé. 12,548 children have suffered a serious adverse event due to the COVID vaccines in the USA; and 106 kids have sadly died.
https://dailyexpose.uk/2022/05/04/children-suffer-due-to-covid-vaccination/

In May 2022, in their court-ordered data document release, Pfizer confessed that 44% of younger subjects experienced "severe" systemic reactions to their vaccine. [146] [It is important to remember that vaccine damage such as myocarditis often does not show up clinically until later; so I suspect the true percentage is much higher.]

Data analyst Jessica Rose traced the tragic case of a 7-year old boy, previously healthy, who died of a cardiac arrest 13 days after his first Pfizer injection. Due to careful record-keeping, Rose was able to trace back the boy's vaccine lot number and searched other adverse events for that specific lot number, which seems to have been targeted to 5 to 11-year old children, and here is that age distribution. [147]

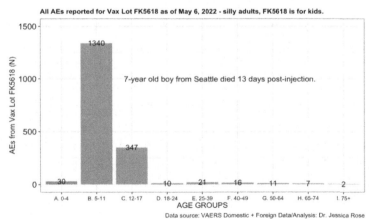

J Rose. Silly adults, this one's for kids. May 9 2022. Substack.
https://jessicar.substack.com/p/silly-adults-this-ones-for-kids

COVID vaccination rates in the US roughly correlate with higher and increasing COVID positivity. Eight of the ten most heavily vaccinated states are at this writing in the top ten highest COVID positivity, as can be seen below. [148] Deaths attributed to COVID-19 do not correlate, but it must be considered that the threshold instructed by the CDC for attributing death to COVID-19 for vaccinated individuals is different than for unvaccinated individuals, or for those vaccinated less than two weeks before death. Therefore, total deaths are a more reliable marker than "COVID-19 deaths."

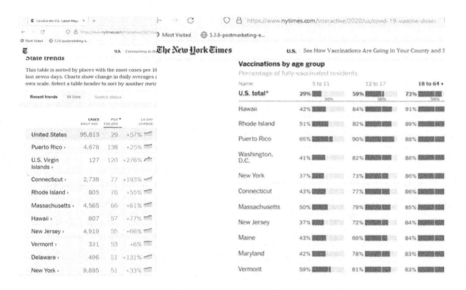

New York Times. Coronavirus in the US . . . May 17 2022.
Graphics © Mapbox and © OpenStreetMap.
https://www.nytimes.com/interactive/2021/us/covid-cases.html

In the UK, COVID-19 deaths are 2 to 3 times as high among the vaccinated as the unvaccinated, according to data analysts at *The Exposé* using official data published by the UK Health Security Agency, shown in the graph below. [149]

The UK government reports tens of thousands of cardiac and hematologic disorders following the Pfizer/BioNTech vaccine alone. [150]

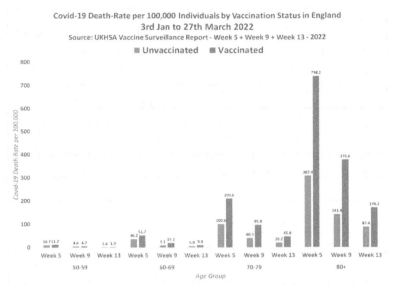

Covid-19 Death-Rate per 100,000 Individuals by Vaccination Status in England
3rd Jan to 27th March 2022
Source: UKHSA Vaccine Surveillance Report - Week 5 + Week 9 + Week 13 - 2022

The Exposé. COVID-19 death rate per 100,000 individuals by vaccination status, Jan 3 to Mar 27 2022. https://dailyexpose.uk/2022/04/27/comparison-gov-reports-proves-vaccinated-suffering-ade/

2) **Consistency** across countries and across continents is observed. It was found in India that the COVID vaccines displayed negative efficacy against Omicron. [151] This is in addition to consistent findings among six other countries in Sections 1 and 4 of these Bradford Hill Criteria. Consistency was also found with the US military: One of the youngest and fittest cohorts in the United States, the military's own recruits, has experienced an 1100% increase in deaths following their mass mandatory vaccination. [152] The medical literature now contains over 1,000 studies regarding injuries and deaths following the COVID vaccines. [153]

Data analysts with The Exposé prepared a visual representation of UK government data, [154] verifiable at UK government documents noted in the following endnotes. The data, all sourced from UKHSA documentation, show negative vaccine efficacy,[155] [156] [157] [158] and is shown here as consistent across all adult age groups:

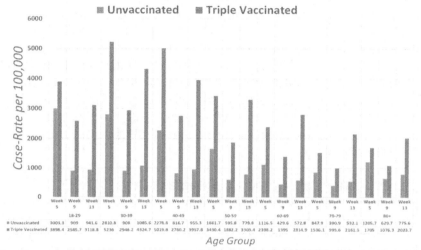

The Exposé, April 28, 2022. https://dailyexpose.uk/2022/04/28/distracted-russia-gov-reveal-triple-jabbed-have-ai-ds/

The weeks selected above, 5, 9 and 13, represent the ends of January, February and March 2022 respectively.

3) **Specificity** is seen in a number of disease and injury conditions as follows. We find higher rates of Omicron among the vaccinated populations of various countries, as in sections 1 and 4 of this chapter, as well as the cardiac injuries discussed in paragraph 6. However, the documents that FDA released under Court order revealed over 1500 types of adverse events observed in the Pfizer trials following the COVID vaccines, which affect all major organ systems. [159] [160] [161] This would argue against specificity; however, we know that it is more common for an environmental toxicant to have a variety of systemic toxic effects, rather than only a specific observed effect in a specific bodily organ.

In the matter of adverse events following the COVID vaccine administration, heart injury, including myocarditis, and neurological injuries and increasing rates of COVID positivity and deaths from these predominate among other reported effects. The cardiovascular injury effect is more specific in that young males are affected more than other demographic groups, according to the CDC. [162] US Health and Human Services Secretary (HHS) Xavier Becerra acknowledged in a White House video session that "We know that vaccines are killing people of color, blacks, Latinos, indigenous people at about two times the rate of white Americans," [163] which seems to be a confession that people of all of those races are being killed by vaccines.

The predominant observed pathologies in the COVID vaccinated have been, and as are supported in this paper, as follows: COVID positivity, with possible immune suppression, cardiovascular injury and deaths from all causes. Secondarily, we see neurological injuries, hepatic injuries and cancers in the COVID-vaccinated, and the latter have fewer supporting studies at this time than the first group, but may all be seen in the Pfizer court-released document referenced above.

4) **Temporality** is seen in Ireland in significantly rising COVID cases following widespread COVID vaccine administration. [164] This was also the case in Germany and South Korea [165] and in Israel for the Delta variant. [166] and in Omicron incidence in Denmark. [167] [168]

A JAMA study of 23.1 million people in national health registers across Scandinavia showed: "The risks of myocarditis and pericarditis were highest within the first 7 days of being vaccinated . . . ." [169]

The VAERS system in the US shows evidence of close temporality. Approximately 50% of deaths occur within the first two days following vaccine administration, as seen in the graph below from Open VAERS, which summarizes VAERS data in a verifiable way. [170] [171]

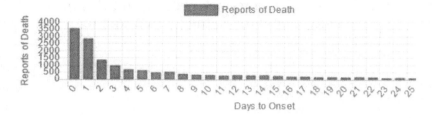

VAERS COVID Vaccine Reports of Deaths by Days to Onset-All Ages

https://openvaers.com/covid-data

The above graph, a compilation of reports to VAERS of deaths following COVID vaccines in the United States by number of days between those events, adheres to a hyperbolic attenuating curve, which further supports cause-effect by temporality. A lack of causation from vaccines to deaths should result in an erratic curve of temporality, without pattern.

The Pfizer lot number described in the first Section of this Chapter, which seems to have been directed to 5 to 11-year old children, shows a very strong temporality signal, in the graph below. [172]

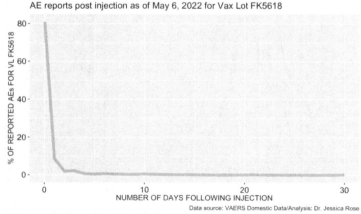

AE reports post injection as of May 6, 2022 for Vax Lot FK5618

Data source: VAERS Domestic Data/Analysis: Dr. Jessica Rose

J Rose. Silly adults, this one's for kids. May 9 2022. Substack.
https://jessicar.substack.com/p/silly-adults-this-ones-for-kids

In Israel there was strong temporal correlation between the 1st and 2nd vaccine doses to young adults, ages 16 to 39 and the number of cardiac arrest emergency calls, as in the graph below. [173] This study appeared in the journal Nature.

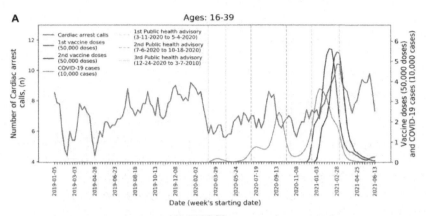

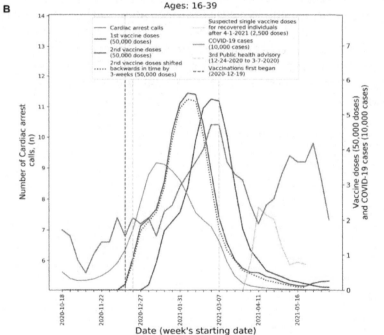

© L Sun, E Jaffe, R Levi. Increased emergency cardiovascular events … Apr 28 2022. Nature Scientific Reports. https://www.nature.com/articles/s41598-022-10928-z#Sec14

The UK government acknowledges close temporality of myocarditis with vaccine dose, "There is an increased risk of myocarditis and pericarditis occurring after vaccination with COVID-19 mRNA vaccine BNT162b2. These conditions can develop within just a few days after vaccination, and have primarily occurred within 14 days." [174]

The above quote from GOV.UK may need to be memorialized in a screenshot, as follows:

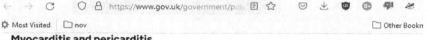

Myocarditis and pericarditis

There is an increased risk of myocarditis and pericarditis occurring after vaccination with COVID-19 mRNA Vaccine BNT162b2. These conditions can develop within just a few days after vaccination, and have primarily occurred within 14 days. They have been observed more often after the second vaccination, and more often in younger males (see section 4.8). Available data suggest that the course of myocarditis and pericarditis following vaccination is not different from myocarditis or pericarditis in general.

Healthcare professionals should be alert to the signs and symptoms of myocarditis and pericarditis. Vaccinated individuals (including parents or caregivers) should also seek immediate medical attention should they experience new onset of chest pain, shortness of breath, palpitations or arrhythmias following vaccination.

The above quote also acknowledges that vaccine-induced myocarditis is not different from myocarditis in general, a disease that results from the permanent death of irreplaceable cells in heart muscle, the very cells that are required to enable the heart to pump blood through the body. I discuss this risk in detail in Chapter 6 of this book.

Myocarditis is an extremely serious disease that has been associated with a 72.4% five-year survival rate. [175]

5) **Biological gradient or dose-response** was seen in the following countries, according to their governments' data:

Case positivity [176] and risk of death were shown to be successively higher with each successive vaccine dose in the UK. [177] [178] [179] Among children ages 10 to 14 in the UK, mortality rates increased substantially with each additional vaccine dose. Children were up to 52 times more likely to die following COVID vaccination than unvaccinated children, as shown in the following graph of data from the Office of National Statistics, UK. [180]

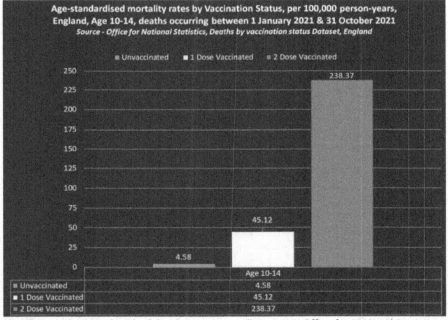

The Exposé. "Children's risk of death increases . . ." From UK Office for National Statistics. Age-standardised mortality rates by vaccination status, per 100,000 person-years, England, Age 10 to 14. Apr 27 2022.
https://dailyexpose.uk/2022/04/27/kids-death-risk-increases-5100percent-covid-vaccination/

In Germany also, the higher the number of vaccines given, the higher the excess mortality. [181]

In the US, Walgreens, one of the two largest pharmacy chains, shows more COVID positivity correlated with more vaccine doses, as shown below. [182]

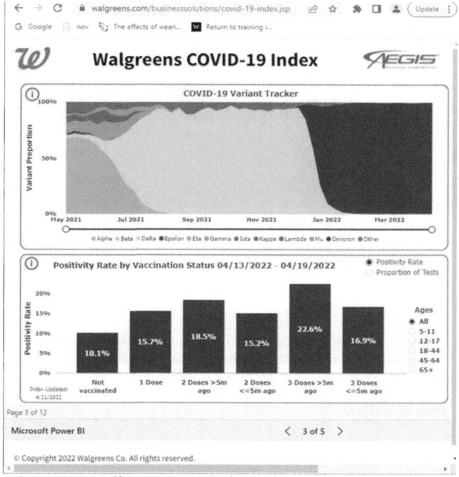

Walgreens.com https://www.walgreens.com/businesssolutions/covid-19-index.jsp

The Government of Canada's official data in the COVID-19 Daily Epidemiology Update shows dose-dependent negative efficacy, consistent with Walgreens' findings above. [183] [184]

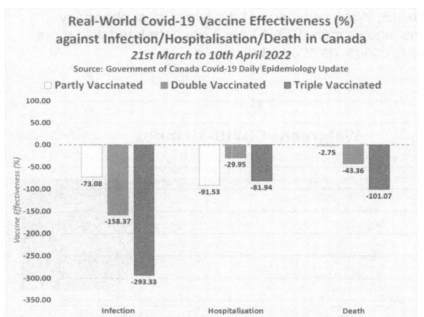

Real-World Covid-19 Vaccine Effectiveness (%)
against Infection/Hospitalisation/Death in Canada
21st March to 10th April 2022
Source: Government of Canada Covid-19 Daily Epidemiology Update

☐ Partly Vaccinated ▪ Double Vaccinated ▪ Triple Vaccinated

The Exposé. Official data suggests the COVID-19 injection is killing more people than it is saving. May 4, 2022. The Exposé.
https://dailyexpose.uk/2022/05/04/covid-vaccine-kills-more-than-it-saves/

Furthermore, higher doses of a single vaccine injection were correlated with more heart damage than lower doses. Specifically, Moderna's vaccine contains 100 micrograms (mcg or µg) of mRNA, whereas Pfizer's vaccine contains 30 mcg of mRNA.

In an enormous study of 23 million Scandinavians, published in the Journal of the American Medical Association, JAMA Cardiology, the Moderna vaccine was correlated with higher rates of myocarditis and pericarditis than the Pfizer vaccine, and the second dose of mRNA vaccine resulted in higher rates of heart damage than only receiving one dose. Each vaccinated group, both Pfizer and Moderna, both single-vaccinated and double-vaccinated, had higher rates of heart damage than unvaccinated people. [185]

The UK government also acknowledges increased risk of myocarditis more often after the second vaccination. [186]

Moderna confessed to the same dangers in their annual SEC filing: "Our vaccine may be associated with higher rates of myocarditis and pericarditis in young males compared to other COVID-19 vaccines. Unexpected safety issues could significantly damage our reputation and that of our mRNA platform . . ." [187]

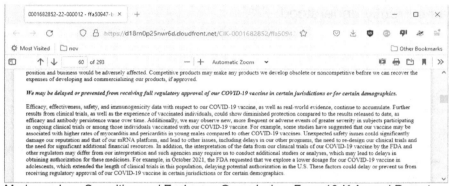

Moderna, Inc. Securities and Exchange Commission. Form 10-K Annual Report Feb 25 2022. P 59. **https://investors.modernatx.com/financials/sec-filings/sec-filings-details/default.aspx?FilingId=15601998**

Myocarditis is considered to be permanently debilitating, and life-shortening, as there is no replacement mechanism for dead cardiomyocytes (the cells that together accomplish the pumping work of the heart). See Chapter 6.

6) **Biological plausibility** for the elevated deaths associated with the COVID vaccines is now theorized. The preponderance of evidence for cardiovascular damage is by means of micro-clotting induced by the mRNA-driven ongoing generation of spike proteins. [188] [189] [190] [191] and that such changes are lasting. [192] [193] [194]

Biological plausibility for the higher rates of Omicron and Delta in vaccinated populations is supported by evidence of damage to the innate and adaptive immune systems, which have been observed to result from these vaccines. [195]

Seneff, Nigh, et al. have outlined observed mechanisms of damage caused by mRNA vaccines, including to innate immunity, especially through damage to our most essential cytokine for fighting viral infections, namely, Type I interferon. Here is their diagram of the scope of mRNA vaccine damage, as currently understood: [196]

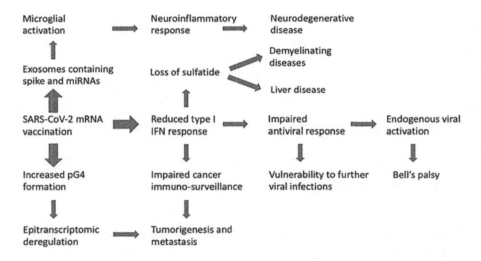

S Seneff, G Nigh, A Kyriakapoulos, P McCullough. Innate immune suppression by SARS-CoV-2 mRNA vaccinations...
https://www.sciencedirect.com/science/article/pii/S027869152200206X

The damage to endogenous interferons leaves the vaccinated more vulnerable to both viruses and cancer, as our innate immunity mechanisms of vigilance against cancer and viruses becomes impaired.

Further evidence of the narrowing of immune effect accomplished by the COVID vaccines is that 93% of unvaccinated first time COVID patients produced antibodies to the nucleocapsid protein (N-protein) of SARS-CoV-2, while only 40% of vaccinated first time COVID patients produced these antibodies. [197] As a result, the vaccinated cohort was rendered with antibodies that were non-neutralizing or fell below a neutralizing level. These are antibodies that are unable to block or clear pathogenic microbes. The result is a limited ability to mount a broad immune response to SARS-CoV-2 virus. This is evidence of an induced vulnerability, and it is one of the bases for warnings of antibody dependent enhancement correlated with the COVID vaccines, as discussed by earlier researchers. [198] and in Chapters 1 and 2.

7) **Coherence** is established by consistency among different ways of analyzing the data. Independent data analysts, using nine different types of analysis, have calculated that the number of Americans killed by the COVID vaccines numbers approximately 388,000, but is at least 150,000. [199] [200]

8) **Experiment** in human populations is unlikely to happen overtly with the COVID vaccines, but self-selecting populations give us an experimental and a control group. In Scotland the unvaccinated had the lowest case rates. [201] The various countries shown in sections 1, 4 and 5 above also compared the vaccinated as an experimental group versus the unvaccinated as a control group, with each self-selected and not randomized.

In this very small, controlled, but not randomized and not blinded study of US high school athletes, control versus experimental groups were established by the athletes' parents' prior choices. None of the vaccinated students complained of fatigue, chest pain or showed declining performance. All of the COVID vaccinated students had some of these symptoms, and all have persistent sports performance deficits compared to their previous performance according to their coaches. [202] This study is the topic of Chapter 5.

Informal reports of widespread cardiac arrest and deaths in athletes have been reported individually, but a pattern of these events has not been acknowledged by governments, sports associations or mainstream media, but have come from several hundred reports from dozens of countries. The actual events of athletes collapsing on fields has been witnessed by millions of sports fans in hundreds of stadiums and fields since early 2021. This article lists each of 942 such events, and for each, the athlete's name, country, date of event and link to the original news article. [203]

9) **Analogy**: Widespread organ damage was seen with previous attempts to use a cationic lipid carrier for mRNA delivery. [204] In this Cell study, whether by intradermal or intramuscular injection, lipid nanoparticles carrying mRNA given to mice were highly inflammatory, with high neutrophil infiltrations, and with "a high mortality rate, with mechanism unresolved." [205]

High mortality has also been observed in animal studies of attempts to vaccinate against coronaviruses. [206] [207]

A brief index of the studies referenced above and listed below in the endnotes may be seen in the following table, organized by application of Bradford Hill criteria. Some studies may be notable in additional categories as well as those listed, and there are many studies not listed here which also address the Bradford Hill criteria, including the over 1,000 NIH studies on Pub Med that support the above data. [208]

Bradford Hill criteria applied to COVID vaccines injuries and deaths			
Studies cited herein, by endnote #	Increase COVID positivity	Cardiovascular injuries	Deaths from all causes
Strength of association	138, 148, 151	139, 146, 147, 150, 169	138, 139, 141-145 149, 152, 153, 181
Consistency	151, 155-158, 164-167, 182-184	140, 159-161	138, 152, 153, 180, 181
Specificity	148, 164-168	162, 169, 174, 187	170, 171
Temporality	164-168	169, 172-174	170, 171
Dose-dependence	176, 182-184	185, 186	138, 177-181
Biological plausibility	195-198	188-194	188 to 194
Coherence	151, 154-158	203	152, 153, 199-200
Experiment	149, 156-158, 201	159, 185, 202, 203	149, 180
Analogy	138, 148, 156-158	204	141, 205-207

Chapter 4

Secondary vaccine effects

The spike protein shedding that Pfizer warned about in their documentation to the FDA seems to have shown up at my clinic. Here is a retrospective study on the data that I collected.

Whereas the primary effects of a medical treatment affect the person receiving the procedure or medication, secondary effects are signs and symptoms in individuals who are close to the patient. Secondary effects are typically of concern, for example, when a cancer patient receives permanent radioactive implants, such as radioactive "seeds." In such cases, pregnant women and small children are generally advised to maintain a distance for two months or to avoid close contact of more than a few minutes.[209] [210]

Primary effects of adverse events following COVID vaccines have been documented at the Vaccine Adverse Event Reporting System (VAERS) of the US Department of Health and Human Services. [211]   Under court order [212] following FOIA request, [213] the FDA released information from the Pfizer data regarding primary adverse events following COVID vaccines, [214] a fraud that exposed the grotesque misplacement of FDA loyalty – to Pfizer, not to the public. The list shows 158,893 "events" following administration of the COVID vaccines. Some of these conditions are known to be permanently disabling and/or life-threatening.

A screenshot of the top part of the first page of that alphabetical list may be seen in Chapter 2.

Secondary effects of the COVID vaccines have been observed in family members and co-workers of people who recently received COVID vaccines. Much of this information has been censored, after informal discussions of these phenomena on social media. [215]

Pfizer had acknowledged to the FDA that spike protein shedding from recently vaccinated people could occur by means of exhalation and skin contact, and that such exposure is "reportable to Pfizer Safety within 24 hours of investigator awareness." [216]

A study of children in vaccinated households compared with children in unvaccinated households showed that the first group had readily detectable SARS-CoV-2 specific IgG antibodies, whereas the latter group lacked those. The effect was stronger when vaccinated parents had high IgG levels. Aerosol transmission of SARS-CoV-2 spike protein from vaccinated person to unvaccinated family members seemed to be the most likely route of transmission, due to consistency with saliva droplets on used facemasks. [217]

A small retrospective study of secondary vaccine side effects

In my naturopathic medical clinic in Arizona, 26 people reported reactions following exposure to COVID vaccinated people, in a time-dependent manner. This was a minority of the patients being currently seen. The following data thus comprise a retrospective case series of patients who reported symptoms after visiting or working with COVID-vaccinated people.

The ages of the affected individuals are from 5 to 80 years, and of both genders, and of multiple races.

The raw data is seen in the table below, in order of month of first exposure, where 1 = January, 2021; 2 = February, 2021, etc.

	Age	Gender	Month of 1st symptoms	From	Symptoms and signs
1	Anonymized data				
2					
3					
4					
5					
6	75	F	1	housemate	spiking hypertension, repeated and marks on skin where touched
7	67	F	1	clients	migraine, malaise, uterine cramping
8	48	F	4	spouse, co-workers	menorrhagia, metrorrhagia
9	78	M	4	wife	fatigue, malaise
10	42	F	4	parents	metrorrhagia, felt "as if uterus and ovaries had been squeezed"
11	37	F	4	restaurant with friends	miscarriage
12	67	F	5	home health care workers	Post-menopausal spotting
13	48	F	5	housemates, cousins	severe menorrhagia --> anemia
14	63	F	5	co-workers	post-men uterine cramping, deranged digestion
15	43	F	5	spouse, family	post-menopausal menorrhagia
16	47	F	5	doctor's office	uterine cramping, menorrhagia
17	60	F	5	MD office	fatigue, night sweats, night agitation
18	5	M	5	grandparents	104 degree fever and seizures, never seized before
19	68	M	5	with friends	hypertension spikes, repeated occurrence
20	63	F	5	hospital work	post-menopausal bleeding
21	63	F	5	patients (3), 7-min exposure	Post-men cramping, bleeding
22	33	M	5	patient, contract worker	flu-like, 2.5 days
23	58	F	6	real estate clients in car	malaise, bloated up to 4 lbs that day, repeated
24	57	F	6	massage tx clients	post-menopausal bleeding, exhaustion, burning hands
25	50	F	6	co-workers	severe menorrhagia, sick, tired, no energy
26	42	M	6	people at a party	fatigue, malaise
27	62	F	6	father	congestion
28	35	F	6	parents	menorrhagia, dysmenorrhea
29	24	F	6	parents	menorrhagia, dysmenorrhea
30	80	F	7	MD office	lymphadenopathy
31	68	M	11	shopping	hypertension spike, first ever
32					

We can see from the above raw data that the preponderance of secondary effects occurred in the spring of 2021, which was a time of high COVID vaccine uptake in the US. That distribution is shown in the following graph:

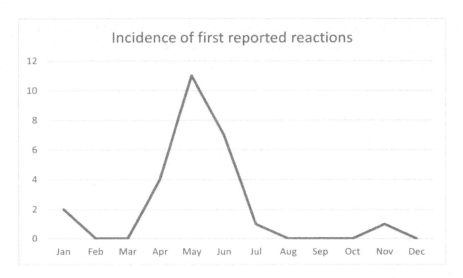

Incidence of first reported reactions

None of the 26 individuals complained of initial reactions from February to March, or from August to October of 2021, nor since December 2021 to the present. This likely corresponds to a time when most of those who wanted COVID vaccines had received them, and then again after boosters were widely available. The one first response in November occurred following a gathering of seniors in which the subject was present. This was a time of known recent booster uptake. One other subject had symptoms near that time, a 68 year old male (line 19) in the first table, who had first had hypertension, which was unusual for him, in June 2021, and then again in December 2021, after booster uptake among those close to him.

Type of symptoms reported:

The following are the major signs and symptoms, and the number of patients with each:
Menstrual irregularities: 7
Post-menopausal menstrual-type symptoms: 6
Miscarriage   1
Fatigue and / or malaise 5
Hypertension   3

Migraine 1
Seizure and fever 1
Lymphadenopathy   1

The preponderance of menstrual symptoms among the signs and symptoms is consistent with known increased concentration of spike proteins in ovaries over other organs. In this study of zebrafish inoculated with spike proteins, a disorganized extracellular matrix in the ovarian stroma was observed. [218]

Treatments

In our clinic, after documenting the reported exposures and signs and symptoms of each individual, we treated them in accordance with a mutually respectful patient-doctor consult culminating in unpressured agreement on appropriate treatment. Patient preference determined which of the following of the doctors' suggestions were followed, and some treatments had been chosen before consult, i.e. ibuprofen, pine needle tea and acetaminophen:

Avoidance 16
Ivermectin 16
N Acetyl Cysteine 12
Pine needle tea   2
Ibuprofen   1
Acetaminophen   1
Vitamin C   1

These add up to more than the 26 patients of the affected cohort, because most chose multiple strategies.   Regarding avoidance, one moved to a very rural area, and has now found relief there; the symptoms had been so intense as to warrant moving from a suburban community.

A retrospective assessment

At this writing, none of the above still report symptoms on questioning, although most have chosen to stop, or to not bother much with, the interventions above. This fast decline in previous symptoms reported, as well as lack of new symptoms reported, and lack of resorting to remedies for the same, suggests that COVID vaccination has not proceeded at such an intense pace following the spring of 2021, and it also suggests that the incidence of spike protein shedding from the vaccinated may have slowed or stopped. Another possibility for the lack of reported symptoms since June 2021 could be habituation or tolerance in the unvaccinated population to spike protein shedding from the vaccinated population.

Chapter 5

Student athletes perform worse than controls following COVID vaccines

I am a co-author on this peer-reviewed article, published on PDMJ.org. Sports coaches had commented to us that vaccinated student athletes were all performing worse than before and than their unvaccinated peers.

Abstract

High school and middle school athletes were observed retrospectively following vaccination with mRNA COVID vaccines. Of twenty student athletes, half were vaccinated and half were not, according to their parents' prior choices. In this study we compare sports performance of vaccinated versus unvaccinated student athletes doing the same activities. We also compare the sports performance of vaccinated student athletes with their own sports performance prior to vaccination. The observed changes post-vaccination can be helpful to illustrate the cardiovascular changes that occur with COVID vaccination.

Introduction

A preponderance of evidence is accumulating with regard to injuries and deaths correlated with the COVID mRNA vaccines. Clinical studies that document this phenomenon now number in the hundreds. [219] Data that was released only under court order from the FDA and Pfizer acknowledged 1,223 deaths and over 1,500 types of adverse events, many of them known to be severely and permanently disabling, with over a total of 158,000 observed adverse reactions, which were found after administration of the Pfizer COVID vaccine, and the reader is encouraged to read the list of these in the last 9 pages of the Pfizer report linked here. [220] This Pfizer document was not made available to the public by the FDA, and the FDA argued that it should be sealed for 55 years, and then for 75 years, but rather it was forced to be released in December 2021 by court order. [221] The overall risks of severe injuries and deaths from the COVID vaccines have alarmed physicians and scientists all over the world. Renowned immunologist and microbiologist Dr. Sucharit Bhakdi and pathologist Dr. Arne Burkhardt have summarized these vaccines' causative role in deaths after vaccination. [222] Autopsy results showed more cardiovascular derangement than for any other organ. Increased inflammatory markers correlate with COVID vaccines. [223] And it is thought that the sudden deaths among athletes during 2021 since the widespread use of the COVID vaccines is mostly due to severe cardiac or cardiovascular pathology.

Methods and Results

Two sports coaches were interviewed regarding performance of their teenage student athletes. On questioning, we learned that there are twenty student athletes with shared training time among the two coaches. Fifteen of these student athletes are high school students, and the rest are younger. The student athletes spoke freely and informally with the coaches about who received the vaccine and how they felt afterward, and who did not receive any vaccines. The student athletes' parents' choices regarding vaccination of their children were unknown to the coaches or to us until after those injections. The parents' choices regarding vaccination of their children had spontaneously formed an experimental group versus a control group, with none blinded.

Strict anonymity is observed regarding the student athletes, their parents, their coaches and their schools, due to the range of emotional responses toward vaccinated and unvaccinated people that has been encouraged over recent months by political leaders such as Joe Biden, Emmanuel Macron and Justin Trudeau.

There was no comparison study of the two groups planned before or at the time of data collection. The two coaches, who spoke to us on condition of anonymity for all involved, retrospectively observed the following of the COVID-vaccinated student athletes, and we report their findings in this retrospective study.

1) None of the vaccinated student athletes are competing up to their own previous level; all are performing worse than in 2020, in the assessments of the two coaches.

2) None of the vaccinated student athletes can endure the same exercise drills for the same amount of time that they used to tolerate prior to vaccination.

3) Recovery from exertion took longer in the vaccinated student athletes than before vaccination and took longer than in the unvaccinated.

4) After the injections, most or all of the vaccinated student athletes talked about one or more of the following reactions after vaccination:

  a) chest pain;
  b) dizziness;
  c) seeing stars;
  d) feeling as if they would faint;
  e) shortness of breath.

The student athletes talked freely and spontaneously about the above symptoms without anyone taking notes at the time. There was no prompting from coaches about reporting of symptoms.

5) The unvaccinated girls are now beating vaccinated boys in competition, whom they could not do well against last year. This change was unexpected and was considered unusual by the coaches.

1), 2), 3) and 5) are still observed in all of the vaccinated student athletes, up to several months after the earliest student athletes were vaccinated.

In contrast, the unvaccinated student athletes had none of the foregoing symptoms or deficits in sports performance or declines in sports endurance, as observed by the two coaches, and continue to improve in their endurance and performance, as expected by the coaches.

Discussion

Athletes may be expected to have more robust circulation during exertion than while sedentary, and generally increased blood flow than is seen in sedentary individuals. Such enhanced circulation, during high activity or exertion serves the purpose of supplying the increased oxygen needs of the body and increased metabolic activity that exertion requires. To increase blood flow requires increased cardiac output and arterial vasodilation. With high cardiac output, there arises increased demand for, and then supply of, coronary arterial blood flow. Coronary arterial vasodilation is regulated by autoregulatory mechanisms, as well as the neurologic vascular innervation mediated by the autonomic nervous system and hormones that serve to adjust vasodilation versus vasoconstriction, as physical activity requires.

The mRNA COVID vaccines begin a process of spike protein production throughout the body. Spike protein effects on ACE 2 receptors in the vascular endothelium serve to vasoconstrict. The result may obstruct the body's supply of increased blood flow and oxygen, just when the demands are greatest, during exertion. Spike protein associated immune and inflammatory factors can also affect perivascular and periarterial cells, as well as CD8 and NK T-cell infiltration. [224] All of these can reduce coronary vasodilation.

Further compounding the problem of blood delivery to peripheral and coronary tissues are the spike protein positions and effects. Jutting from the endothelial surface, spike proteins are docked onto ACE-2 receptors. These are thought to adversely affect blood flow through turbulent rather than laminar flow. As stagnant blood pools, the clotting cascade begins ubiquitously throughout the body. Such micro-clotting thickens and slows the blood, which would further impair the delivery of blood and oxygen to the capillary beds in the heart and in the periphery. Thus, coronary blood flow can be adversely affected by high viscosity, which is also caused by spike protein-induced RBC aggregation from adhesion through CD 147. As a result, the heart is burdened to push a more viscous liquid than normal blood through the body's arterioles and capillaries.

The above-described mechanisms, further described here, [225] create obstacles to optimal blood flow that would necessarily affect all recipients of spike protein generating COVID vaccines. We therefore must recommend avoidance of any of the COVID vaccines by any child or young adult with current or future plans to engage in physical exertion.

Mechanisms of Risk

Chapter 6

Heart damage from the COVID vaccines: Is it avoidable?

Or do all COVID-vaccinated people have some myocarditis?

Abstract

This paper addresses the question of prevalence of COVID vaccine-associated myocarditis, as well as known mechanisms of spike protein-induced myocarditis, considering the epidemiological consequences of mass vaccination with spike protein-generating COVID vaccines, such as are being deployed throughout the world at present. The cardiac impacts of spike protein distribution have risen to particular concern, due to the recent extraordinary increase in new cases of myocarditis and pericarditis, including among populations that typically have vanishingly rare incidence of this disease, especially young men, with particularly anomalous occurrence in young male athletes.

Introduction

The US Centers for Disease Control and Prevention (CDC) finds increased reported cases of myocarditis and pericarditis following mRNA COVID-19 vaccination, most notably in adolescents and young adults, [226] including in the absence of COVID-19 infection. [227] Myocarditis was only rarely found post-vaccination prior to the COVID mRNA vaccines, and then mostly associated with the smallpox vaccine. [228] Typically and historically, myocarditis patients are older with high prevalence of diabetes, hypertension, atrial fibrillation, coronary artery disease and heart failure. [229] Myocarditis is an extremely concerning condition. At five years post-diagnosis, myocardial injury, which is a clinically indistinguishable condition from myocarditis, and is often discussed interchangeably and synonymously, is correlated with a 72.4% mortality rate, and is therefore correlated with higher mortality than even Type 1 myocardial infarction (rupture of coronary artery plaque with thrombus) or Type 2 myocardial infarction (vasospasm generally), which have 36.7% and 62.5% five-year mortality rates respectively. [230] So myocarditis is likely even more concerning than myocardial infarction. This may be due to the generalized cytotoxic injury, due to external cause, throughout the heart in the myocarditis event, compared to the localized watershed damage affecting a portion of the heart, which is associated with myocardial infarction.

Heart function is mostly regulated by cardiomyocytes and vascular endothelial cells. Cardiomyocytes have no potential for self-renewal, as they are terminally differentiated cells. When they die, they necrose and are replaced by proliferating fibroblasts, which form fibrotic tissue. This tissue reduces systolic function, and is associated with a poor prognosis. [231]

Due to the generally much higher activity level of a young athlete than of the historical prototype myocarditis patient, are we simply noticing greater contrast in activity level before and after the COVID vaccines in the former, and missing this contrast, and hence the myocarditis diagnosis, in more sedentary individuals? This paper will examine the possible mechanisms of the mRNA COVID vaccine association with myocarditis, in order to assess how common this association might be.

When asked in June 2021 about the risk of myocarditis following the COVID vaccines, Dr. Roger Hodkinson, pathologist, replied:

> *"Myocarditis is never mild, particularly in young healthy males. It's an inflammation of the heart muscle, the pump of the body. And we don't know what percent of the heart muscle cells would have died in any one attack of myocarditis. The big thing about heart muscle, heart muscle fibers, is that they do not regenerate, . . . so you're stuck with an unknown percentage of your heart muscle cells having died. We can't estimate the number, and therefore the long-term results are utterly unpredictable. We do know . . . that myocarditis can present decades later, with premature onset of heart failure that would otherwise not have been expected. So it's a terrible worry for these people to know what's going to happen to them in the future. . . . It's not trivial."* [232]

When asked in April 2022 about the risk of myocarditis following the COVID vaccines, Dr. Peter McCullough, cardiologist and medical journal editor said:

> *"The spike protein is super thrombogenic and makes all clot risk scenarios worse."* [233] *. . . . Myocarditis is of great concern in male athletes and military where surges in adrenaline superimposed on spike protein subclinical myocardial damage triggers cardiac death in the susceptible. In some it's too late for CPR.* [234]

In diagnosing myocarditis, cardiac magnetic resonance studies (CMR) have shown specific sites of inflammation or fibrosis, and help to evaluate functional impairment of heart muscle. Myocardial edema and late gadolinium enhancement are seen on CMR in cases of myocarditis. In all cases reporting chest pain post-COVID vaccine in one study these abnormal findings were present on CMR in each subject. Past or current COVID-19 disease had been excluded in all subjects. [235] However, the more widely accepted criterion of myocardial injury is a threshold of serum troponin levels at or above 99th percentile of upper reference range. [236] Elevated troponin is considered to be both sensitive and specific for myocardial damage. Troponin is a protein normally confined to the cytosol of cardiomyocytes, as well as other muscle cells, and is not normally found in the blood; however, it is released in the circulation when heart muscle cells become damaged.

At the time of this writing, in the current post-peak-COVID era, it has been 15 months since peak COVID mortality in the US and the world, which occurred in mid-April 2020, as shown by CDC data. [237] Now, a year later, COVID vaccines have been aggressively introduced in most countries, and Our World In Data, which is funded by the Bill and Melinda Gates Foundation, estimates that 2.5 billion people or one quarter of the earth's population, have already taken one of the new COVID vaccines, although they have only been available for about six months. [238] As morbidity and mortality from SARS-CoV-2 and COVID-19 and its variants have diminished, and the world's death rate per 1000 people is still at a relative low in 2020 and 2021 compared to the last seven decades, without evidence of any recent pandemic by mortality data, [239] we now can turn our attention to the health effects of the new COVID vaccines. None of the new vaccines attempts to introduce the entire coronavirus into the body, but rather a spike protein generating mechanism. Therefore, let's focus on only the spike protein's effects on the myocardium and its cells.

Mechanisms

Recent introduction of mRNA vaccines that program human cells' genetic mechanisms to generate spike proteins has led to an increased interface generally between spike proteins and bodily tissues. These recently increased venues of interaction have apparently exceeded, both in human populations and in human tissues, the levels that mRNA vaccine developers had expected. For unknown reasons, mRNA vaccine developers had expected spike proteins to remain entirely in the deltoid muscle at the vaccination site of the vaccinated person, as reported in the media, [240] and it was apparently imagined – contrary to basic circulatory physiology – that these spike proteins could somehow evade both lymphatic drainage and release into the general circulation.

However, it has recently been determined that the delivery of spike proteins and / or their generating mechanisms, as with all known injected substances, do indeed diffuse and travel in an organism, away from the site of injection, in accordance with well-established principles of circulation, throughout the body, including to internal organs. Organs that have been affected by this body-wide distribution have included the heart, brain, spleen and liver, with especially high concentrations found in the ovaries and the plasma. [241]

The spike protein is the part of coronaviruses in general, and SARS-CoV-2 in particular, that attaches to and interacts with human cell membranes. I examine the role of the SARS-CoV-2 spike protein on the myocardium, and mechanisms by which the cardiomyocytes and vascular endothelial cells, which predominate there, may be threatened by such exposure. It is possible that other elements of the SARS-CoV-2 virus, besides spike proteins, have deleterious effects on cells, including risk for myocarditis. [242]

It has been observed also that mRNA interventions are fragile and unpredictable in their effect,[243] and have been seen to damage mitochondria by a number of known mechanisms.[244] Of patients hospitalized for COVID-19, myocarditis-pattern injury was observed in 4.5%[245] to 27% of cases.[246] Moreover, in the event of SARS-CoV-2 infection, it was found that the associated cytotoxic and pro-apoptotic effects were sufficient to abolish cardiomyocyte beating (contraction-relaxation cycles).[247] However, direct virus replication was not found on examination of the myocardium, [248] [249] and SARS-CoV-2 RNA was not found in the cardiomyocytes. [250] Therefore, it is worthwhile to examine if post-vaccine myocarditis is likely to be caused by spike proteins generated by the vaccines, and to result from either the cytokine storm or from the endothelial damage caused by spike proteins. Considering a wider set of possible causes, we know that fulminant SARS-CoV-2 infection is characterized by hypoxia, systemic inflammation, and possibly thrombosis and / or cardiomyopathy, and even the possibility of myocarditis. All of these have been observed *in vitro* in the presence of spike proteins, and all of these can result in higher levels of measured troponin, which in turn establishes diagnosis of myocarditis, or at least clinical awareness of signs of myocarditis. [251]

At this time, there is not any other part of the SARS-CoV-2 virus that is known to attach to human cells. The binding of the spike protein to cell membranes initiates a cascade of events that result in fusion of the viral and cellular membranes and entry of the virus into the human cytoplasm. [252] Most of this activity in most human cells seems to involve one or both of the S1 subunits of the spike protein, but for human brain endothelial cells, it seems the S2 subunit of the spike protein is involved. [253] Human host cell proteases participate in this fusion and entry. [254]

The spike proteins that are generated by the mRNA COVID vaccines are said to be identical to those attached to SARS-CoV-2. [255] The spike protein in SARS-CoV-2 is a trimeric, or three-part protein, composed of two functional S1 subunits, as well as a structural S2 subunit. Each of those three units are, incidentally, bound and inactivated by the drug ivermectin. [256] In the absence of ivermectin or hydroxychloroquine, the two drugs most thoroughly studied and most widely used in early and late cases of COVID-19, [257] the spike protein remains in a conformation that enables it to attach to the ACE2 receptor on human cells, and to enter by that portal. Conversely, either of those drugs is able to change the conformation of the spike protein in such a way that prevents entry to the human cell. [258]

ACE2 receptors are found in cells throughout the human body, and have been shown to have varying effects on different organs. ACE2 receptors have been found to be highly concentrated in cardiac pericytes, [259] even more so than in the lungs. [260] But the presence of ACE2 has been observed to have a seemingly paradoxical protective effect in the cardiovascular system, such as preserving ATP production. [261] Spike proteins have been found to down-regulate ACE2. [262] Human cardiomyocytes have been observed to express the ACE2 receptor, and that is the main portal by which the spike protein of SARS-CoV-2 is observed to attach. In addition to the ACE2 receptor, the CD-147 receptor is also used by the spike protein to enter host cells. [263]

Spike protein was found to enter cardiomyocytes *in vitro*, and cytotoxicity was detected at 24 hours post exposure, and "profound cytopathogenic effects" were visible at 96 hours in cardiomyocytes. [264]

The spike protein alone of SARS-CoV-2 has been found to have damaging effects on endothelial function. [265] In fact, the spike protein alone was found to produce pro-apoptotic factors that were determined by researchers to be responsible for endothelial cell death. [266] Endothelial cells that were treated with the spike protein showed mitochondrial fragmentation and dysmorphic changes, as well as reduced mitochondrial respiration with redox stress, but increased glycolysis, and it was shown that the S protein alone damaged endothelial cells by this mechanism. [267] Interestingly, in those *in vitro* studies, cell function was found to be restored by adding N-acetyl-L-cysteine, which is a reactive oxygen species inhibitor.

The spike protein has been found, without other viral elements, to stimulate cell signaling in human cardiac pericytes that has been associated with cardiac cell dysfunction. Some of this dysfunction includes findings of increased amounts of the following pro-inflammatory cytokines (those involved in cytokine storms) in cardiac pericytes on *in vitro* exposure to S protein: MCP-1, IL-6, IL-1B and TNF-alpha.[268] TNF-alpha is specifically associated with heart failure and myocarditis. [269]

Caspase-3 is associated with apoptosis. When coronary artery endothelial cells were exposed to spike protein, they were found to have increased Caspase-3/7 activity, which was correlated with pro-apoptotic effect. Some of the above activity was through the ACE-2 receptor, but more data showed involvement of the CD-147 receptor on those cells, [270] and we have seen above that both pathways are used by spike proteins for cell entry. The cell death experienced in myocarditis seems likely to be at least partly due to this activity.

Electrocardiogram (EKG) abnormalities have also been found following COVID vaccine administration. This includes diffuse ST elevation and an inverted T-wave in lead III, as well as sinus tachycardia. [271]

A summary of expected effects after COVID vaccination is in Figure 1.

Figure 1: Cardiovascular events following COVID vaccination

Spike protein enters circulation	→	attaches to ACE2 and CD147 receptors	→	enters endothelial cells		↗ caspase protein And mitochondrial damage	→	apoptosis
				↘ and pericytes		↗ pro-inflammatory cytokines	→	inflammation
				↘ and cardiomyocytes				

↓

Damaged and dysfunctional mitochondria, And loss of beating, And profound cytopathogenic effects within 96 hours

↓

Cardiomyocyte death

↓

Irreversible myocarditis

Discussion

The pathways discussed herein are inevitable routes of spike protein transit in the body and in the cells. ACE2 receptors are abundant in every known cell type. When spike proteins have been introduced to the body, either through the SARS-CoV-2 virus or by means of the mRNA COVID vaccines, is there any realistic way possible to block their interaction with ACE2 receptors in any individual? In the case of acute infection with SARS-CoV-2, infected individuals have a self-limiting encounter with spike proteins, which may be thwarted by some of the therapeutics mentioned above. However, in the case of the mRNA-vaccinated, no endpoint of spike protein production is yet known. Nor is it yet known if it is safe to use any of the spike protein-blocking therapeutics in vaccinated individuals.

In the absence of extraordinary and deliberate measures to block ACE2 receptors and CD147 receptors and/or Caspase 3/7 activity, is it then possible to expect that cardiac pericytes and endothelial cells could escape the pro-inflammatory and pro-apoptotic effects of the spike protein, especially considering that protein's perpetual regeneration in vaccinated people? Could a therapeutic be invented for vaccinated people to protect their cardiomyocytes and pericytes from spike protein damage, and to be dosed frequently enough to combat the body's ongoing spike protein production? If such an expectation is not realistic, then mRNA vaccines that prepare human cells to generate an unknown supply of spike proteins for an unknown amount of time are to be treated with extreme caution and avoidance until better understood.

Dr. Peter McCullough is the most widely published cardiologist in human history. He has warned tirelessly of cardiovascular and hematologic damage from the COVID vaccines, and he also warns of the cumulative risk of successive vaccines continually producing spike proteins without a known endpoint to that production of toxins. [272]

It is also necessary to defer further vaccination until there are known methods of both discharge of such proteins and the mechanism to turn off or attenuate mRNA-induced spike proteins, and/or to safely thwart the destructive effects of spike proteins in host cells.

We must also urgently learn the answer to the following question: Is the human recipient of a spike protein-generating mRNA vaccine reasonably expected to continue to generate spike proteins for an indefinite amount of time? Or even permanently? We need to know this, because the spike protein has been shown to have deleterious effects, and because myocarditis, which seems to be one of those effects, is now being observed in some vaccinated individuals, the mechanisms of which are discussed in this paper.

There is observed precedent for mRNA medical treatments to have lasting effect on DNA, [273] [274] [275] [276] which impacts future as well as present generations. Questions involving such serious potential consequences for human health must be answered, and standards of safety and informed consent must be met, before an ambitious and experimental procedure on the massive scale we are witnessing is deployed on populations. As a result, vaccines of this type must be avoided until these questions are thoroughly resolved, in order to prevent further harm to human health.

Chapter 7

Heart fatigue from vaccines, as shown by fluid dynamics

Blowing water out of a straw is easy, right?
What if it were milk instead? No problem.
What if it were maple syrup? What if your heart
were challenged to make a similar effort 24 / 7 ?

The path of blood from the heart through the body's circulatory system takes blood, its cells and dissolved nutrients through a path from wide to narrow to wide again. This happens when the blood, pumped from the left ventricle of the heart, flows through the wide aorta (our body's main central artery), and is then pushed through ever-narrower arteries. Then in turn, these branch into narrower arterioles, and finally into the capillaries. The capillaries are so small, so thin, that even a microscopic red blood cell must fold and momentarily deform a bit, in order to make it through that tunnel in order to get some elbow room, so to speak, on to a venule, then a vein, and then to the spacious vena cava (our body's central vein) in its perpetual round trip journey back to the heart.

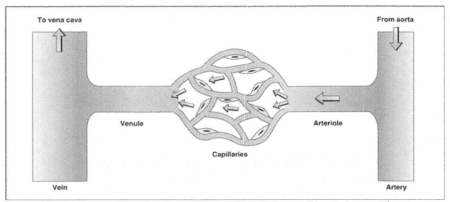

From *Hemodynamics, Cardiovascular Physiology, Physiology, 5th ed.*

When blood is normally thin, this journey has little resistance – even with narrowing vessels, because there are an increasing number of those vessels on roughly parallel paths, dividing the flow of blood. Blood pressure stays low to moderate, and the heart does not have to work particularly hard to move blood around.

But blood is not always thin these days. The cardiovascular effects of the COVID vaccines are comparable to placing many rocks in the creek, so to speak, which in an actual creek would change smooth flow to turbulence, stagnant eddies here, and rapids there.

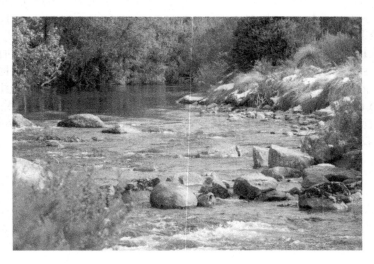

The mRNA vaccines deliver an estimated 40 trillion packets of mRNA instruction code for human cells to produce spike proteins. The "spikes" are well-named, because when they are released from the cells where they are produced, and then into the bloodstream and come to dock at the ACE-2 and CD-147 receptors, their shape disrupts the smooth surface of the inner lining of the blood vessel.

Once laminar smooth blood flow now becomes disrupted by turbulence and momentary stagnation, which immediately leads to clotting. But none of these are large injuries, so the phenomenon is a widespread micro-clotting and a general viscosity of blood.

Angeli and Spanevello, et al, discuss the problem that results after human cells are targeted and destroyed by vaccines, and then release spike proteins. Then these spike proteins interact with ACE-2 receptors on other cells, which promotes ACE-2 internalization and degradation into lysosomes. [277] [278] This docking of spike proteins on human cells' ACE-2 receptors has been shown to promote platelet aggregation. [279]

The mRNA instruction to human cells is to produce and release spike proteins from cells, to then float freely until the spike proteins dock onto the endothelial cells lining blood vessels and jut out into the lumen, just as boulders jut into the flowing water of a stream, changing the water's motion.

There are also CD-147 receptors and the effects of spike protein attachment there, as well as other considerations of endothelial cell death, inflammation associated with spike proteins, as well as the activity of platelets in the newly formed microclots. I discuss these mechanisms more elsewhere. [280]

How thick blood flows

As a stream of fluid (liquid or gas) is forced by the pumping of the heart against a constricted opening, both its speed (v) and kinetic energy (KE) increase. Bernoulli's equation explains the physics principle of conservation of energy, in the specific case of a fluid being forced through a narrowed opening:

$$\frac{1}{2}\rho v^2 = \frac{\frac{1}{2}mv^2}{V} = \frac{KE}{V}$$

Where ρ is the fluid density, and the kinetic energy per unit volume KE/V is ½ of mass times the square of velocity per total Volume (V). But don't worry about that so much. More importantly, Bernoulli's equation tells us that if there is something that raises the viscosity of blood, then there is a corresponding rise in the kinetic energy expended to move blood around. According to Bernoulli's equation above, the increased fluid density corresponds to a rise in energy used in moving blood through vessels. This would create more effort for the heart. We know from decades of experience with atherosclerotic patients, that when the heart labors to push blood through rigid blood vessels that cannot dilate well, then not only does blood pressure rise, but the overworked heart is at risk of congestive heart failure, which is a concerning disease that has a 30% survival rate a decade after diagnosis.

Resistance in the cardiovascular system is directly proportional to blood viscosity, where η is the viscosity of blood. (With a fluid, the tactile sensation of "viscosity" or thickness of a liquid, is quantified by osmolarity, often in mOsm/L. Osmolarity is just a quantifiable way of assessing viscosity.)

There is a further consideration with having viscous blood. The symbol π_c represents capillary oncotic pressure, which means an inward pressure or the tendency to draw fluid inward. When π_c increases, such as when blood is thickened by the involved process of conglomeration of various microclot components, then the plasma part of blood may tend to stay in the capillaries and not diffuse into the surrounding tissues. This would have the effect of increasing blood pressure, until other homeostatic mechanisms take effect.

Here is a corollary of Poiseuille's equation, in which resistance (or the drudgery of pushing thick blood through the body) is proportional to the blood's viscosity and to the length of the vessels, but is inversely related to the radius of the vessels.

$$R = \frac{8\eta L}{\pi r^4}$$

So let's say you got the COVID vaccine(s), but you still want to be able to have your heart push blood easily around your body. The above equation shows that resistance (R) increases when length (L) increases. This means that you have to blow water harder out through a very long straw than through a short straw. But resistance also increases when viscosity (η, pronounced EE-ta) increases. So you have more difficulty blowing maple syrup through a straw than water through a straw. The denominator of the equation gives a way out of the dilemma of COVID vaccine-induced viscosity creating extra resistance. The radius of the blood vessel is r. In Poiseuille's equation, we see that r is in the denominator, so if the radius (or rather, r^4) increases, then you can have lower resistance again. So vasodilation may be a strategy that clinicians explore if COVID vaccinated patients develop hypertension.

It's possible that the problem of a chronically overworked heart could be medicated with positive inotropic agents, which boost heart-pumping force, such as digoxin, but this may lead to pump burnout (heart failure) in the nearer term. So other strategies could possibly include various ways to lower blood pressure by vasodilation or by means of beta-blockers, ACE inhibitors and angiotensin receptor-blocking drugs.

The most widely published cardiologist in human history is Peter McCullough MD. Dr. McCullough urges the appreciation of heart muscle:

> *"In cardiology we spend our entire career trying to save every bit of heart muscle. We put in stents, we do heart catheterization, we do stress tests, we do CT angiograms. The whole game of cardiology is to preserve heart muscle. Under no circumstances would we accept a vaccine that causes even one person to sustain heart damage. Not one. . . . for some other theoretical benefit for a viral infection, which for most is less than a common cold, is untenable. The benefits of the vaccines in no way outweigh the risks."*

As an abundance of caution, it is important to not use any of the currently available COVID vaccines with either children or adults, until the cardiovascular consequences are better understood, or for those who are already vaccinated, to offer therapies that are appropriate for the cardiovascular consequences that patients present clinically. [281]

How can you know if you or a loved one has suffered a cardiovascular injury following a vaccine? Dr.McCullough says: "People need to be paying attention to their symptoms . . . . They have to pay attention to leg pain, swelling, chest pain, signs and symptoms . . . People need an evaluation. The same thing is true for headaches.. . . ." [282]

Are All Vaccines Hazardous?

Chapter 8

What is in a vaccine?

Vaccine adjuvants, their role, and
risk mitigation if you spill such
substances on your skin or elsewhere

Adjuvants are substances that have been added to vaccines
for about a century, and that are present in every vaccine that
is commercially produced. Their alleged purpose is to
enhance the immune response. Adjuvant is from the Latin
adjuvare (to aid). In fact, they are substances that are each
documented in chemical industry literature to have shown
concerning effects on exposure. The standard toxicology
reference documents in the chemical industry are the Oxford
Materials Safety Data Sheets, and I reference those in the
tables below.

Why would known poisons be added to vaccines? One may
speculate on a variety of motives for their presence, but the
official explanation is basically this:

The mechanism of adding a small amount of a poison to a tool
that is hoped to stimulate immune function is that by means of
some cell death, metabolic disruption and / or tissue damage,
the whole immune system is placed on high alert to muster its
forces to wage war against the new crisis: the new poison
introduced by breach of skin and mucous membrane armor.

Table 1:
Common adjuvants currently used in common childhood vaccines and emergency measures to use in case of exposure

Adjuvants used in licensed vaccines [283]	Components	Instructions for mitigating risks of exposure listed in the Oxford Material Safety Data Sheets [284]
Alum	Aluminum hydroxide	Irritant to eyes and skin; "serious eye damage"
	Aluminum phosphate	If inhaled or ingested, get medical attention. For skin or eye contact, rinse immediately with plenty of water for 15 minutes.
MF59		
	Squalene	If in eyes, rinse thoroughly with plenty of water for 15 minutes. Ensure adequate ventilation.
	Tween (polysorbate) 80	If swallowed, make victim drink water (two glasses at least). In case of skin contact, take off immediately all contaminated clothing. Rinse skin with water/shower. In case of eye contact, rinse out with plenty of water. Use PPE with gloves, minimum layer thickness: 0.11 mm
	Span 85 (Sorbitan trioleate)	If breathed in, move person into fresh air. In case of skin contact, wash off with soap and plenty of water.
AS04		
	Alum	See above for alum ingredients
	MPL (monophosphoryl lipid A)	Pyrogen derived from Salmonella. If breathed in, move person into fresh air. In case of skin contact, wash off with soap and plenty of water.
AS03		
	Squalene with alpha-tocopherol	See above for squalene
	Tween (polysorbate) 80	See above for Tween
AS01		
	MPL (monophosphoryl lipid A)	See above for MPL
	QS-21	Hemolysis of red blood cells [285]
	Liposomes	[presumed delivery system]
CpG 1018		
	22-mer single-stranded DNA	[exogenous DNA]

Table 2:
Adjuvants used in COVID vaccines for adults and emergency measures to use in case of exposure

Adjuvants in COVID vaccines [286]	Toxic effects from Oxford Material Safety Data Sheets [287]
Polyethylene glycol	If inhaled, remove to fresh air. If ingested, clean mouth with water and drink afterwards plenty of water. If skin or eye contact, rinse immediately with plenty of water for at least 15 minutes. Seek medical attention. Handler with PPE. Ensure adequate ventilation. Avoid contact with skin, eyes or clothing.
	Anaphylactic shock [288]
Cationic lipids	Damage to lungs, mitochondria, red blood cells, white blood cells, liver, nervous system [289] [290]

Table 3:
Adjuvant proposed for use in COVID vaccines for 5-11 years of age and emergency measures to use in case of exposure

Proposed adjuvant to be used in COVID vaccines for children [291]	Toxic effects from Oxford Material Safety Data Sheets [292]
Tromethamine (Common name "Tris")	If inhaled, remove to fresh air. If ingested, clean mouth with water and drink afterwards plenty of water. If skin or eye contact, rinse immediately with plenty of water for at least 15 minutes. Seek medical attention. Handler with PPE. Ensure adequate ventilation. Avoid contact with skin, eyes or clothing.

Tromethamine (or "Tris" or "Tham") is a blood acid reducer that can reduce acid levels in the body following heart surgery or cardiac arrest. Now why would such a substance need to be added to the COVID vaccine? Could it be that a new epidemic of heart disease is being caused by these vaccines in the older age groups? Indeed, we are seeing increased hospitalization around the world, only partially but not mostly attributed to COVID, since widespread COVID vaccine distribution.

The adjuvant method of using a small dose poison to "aid" or to elicit a systemic reaction, although widely upheld as a necessary aspect of exemplary scientific practice by vaccine enthusiasts, has been widely and vehemently rejected when applied homeopathically, as for example when 18th century physician Samuel Hahnemann dosed himself orally with small doses of quinine from the bark of cinchona trees, which simulated malaria symptoms, and then seemed to have protective effect against malaria.   Since then, homeopaths have even treated with minute (even below Avogadro's number) amounts of arsenic, strychnine and other poisons, in order to alert the hypothalamus to restore homeostasis, to overcome symptoms and illness.   But homeopathy has never had lobbyists in the US Congress, so never mind about that.

The adjuvant substances listed above should give rise to concern among the public and the health care professions regarding their use, and should draw particular attention to the requirement for informed consent, as mandated under the Code of Federal Regulations: 45 CFR § 46.116, particularly section (a), (b), with particular attention to (b) (8), (c) and (i).

The Occupational Safety and Health Administration (OSHA) has been asked by the Biden Administration to force vaccination in US workplaces, first large and possibly small businesses also. However, Congress established OSHA's toxicology standard, as upheld by the Supreme Court, to be: "Standard which most adequately assures, to the extent feasible, on the basis of best available evidence, that no employee will suffer material impairment of health or functional capacity even if such employee has regular exposure to the hazard dealt with by such a standard for the period of his working life." [293] The OSHA standards for chemical exposures then have been established as **_maximum_** permissible exposure to substances, not **_minimum_** permissible exposure. This alone disqualifies OSHA from mandating the introduction of a new hazard that is not desired by either employer or employees. And therefore, the Biden mandates are null and void, because they are pre-empted by existing laws and federal regulations regarding OSHA's role in the workplace.

The issue of informed consent has a history in the massively devastating and painful lesson of the Holocaust: that medical procedures must never be forced on individuals. It is enshrined in the Nuremberg Code, the Universal Declaration of Human Rights, the Geneva Medical Declaration as well as United States law. Have the vaccinators in your midst ensured that your "refusal to participate will involve no penalty or loss of benefits to which the subject is otherwise entitled, and the subject may discontinue participation at any time without penalty or loss of benefits to which the subject is otherwise entitled?" [294]

Have the vaccinators in your midst acknowledged the experimental nature of the COVID vaccines, and that as the public participates in the Phase 3 trials of the COVID vaccines without being so informed, also contrary to informed consent law, the COVID-vaccinated people are *de facto* research subjects? Have the vaccinators in your midst made you aware of any of the above risk mitigation recommendations for the adjuvants they propose to inject into you?

Consider the enormous increase in miscarriages discussed above in Chapters 1 and 2, and the ubiquitous urging and bullying of pregnant women to be vaccinated. Nearly a year after the shot had first been pushed on pregnant women, the FDA stated that proper information for use in pregnant and nursing women is missing:

> "Missing information: Use in pregnancy and lactation; Vaccine effectiveness; Use in pediatric individuals <12 years of age." [295] [296]

"In the early Renaissance, the Italians . . . brought the art of poisoning to its zenith. The poisoner became an integral part of the political scene. The records of the city councils of Florence . . . contain ample testimony about the political use of poisons. Victims were named, prices set, and contracts recorded; when the deed was accomplished, payment was made." [297]

Chapter 9

Immunology 101.1

Vaccines target a small portion of the entire human immune system, and often lag behind mutations of microbes. Yet vaccines have dazzled humans for centuries.

"The best vaccination is to get infected yourself.
And if she really has the flu,
she definitely doesn't need the flu vaccine."

Dr. Anthony Fauci, C-SPAN, October 11, 2004 [298]

Let's consider the vastness of the human immune system, the resource that the body utilizes in encounters with any virus or other invading microbe. This essay gets a bit into the weeds of human immune function and will seem as esoteric on first encounter as it does to first year medical students. I summarize below the complex and synchronized activities of the vast majority of immune players that are at work and what they accomplish together, before the small remainder, the object of vaccine activity, namely B-cells and the antibodies made by them, even show up.

There are two branches of the immune system in humans. These are the innate and the adaptive immune systems. Vaccines target about five percent of immune system cells, namely B-cells, and although some would argue T-cells also, any evidence for that is much weaker and not widely considered to be credible. The innate immune system, which does not make any demonstrated beneficial use of vaccines, is the older of the two, the more widespread in the animal kingdom, and the one that has been active in our bodies since birth.

Considering first the innate immune system, the larger and far more versatile of the two major branches, it is so ubiquitous throughout the body that cells of the innate immune system are no farther from any other cell in the body than the thickness of a fingernail. This short distance represents the maximum distance of any living cell to the nearest capillary blood vessel that nourishes it. When you get a "complete blood count" from your lab, and you see neutrophils, monocytes, etc., you are looking at counts of cells per milliliter (or microliter, as indicated) of liquid blood that move through every blood vessel. The innate immune system has the larger share of cells in the blood, many more than the adaptive immune system.

Although cells are basic units of the immune system, the epithelial barriers of the skin and mucous membranes are the first defenses involved in innate immunity. These function best when they are intact barriers. When those barriers are not abraded, lacerated or punctured, they are better able to exclude invading pathogens, which are microscopic infectious agents, from the far more vulnerable internal tissues and organs. The skin is more visible than the mucous membranes, but there's not as much of it -- 2 square meters versus 400 square meters for the latter, or the size of two tennis courts. How is the latter so large in just one person's body? Think of all the folds and turns of the intestinal villi and the respiratory epithelia.

The skin is our ultimate shield against the abundant microbial world just outside it. Vaccines are Trojan horse mechanisms that, among other effects, breach and defeat the strongest purpose of our very advanced and formidable yet supple armor.

Our innate immune system continues beneath the surface. It is the tapestry of the paths of first responding cells that are ready everywhere to attack invading pathogens (from a splinter, insect sting, just inhaled microbes, etc.) In fact, this level of vigilance is so comprehensive throughout the body, that very often new pathogens are completely defeated and dispatched, even weeks before the antibodies of the adaptive immune system would begin to ramp up activity. The various types of cells in the innate immune system are the tools that the body calls on to destroy invading pathogens.

Macrophages (literally *big eaters*) have been just under the skin everywhere throughout the body since birth, mainly cleaning up the debris of cellular processes, such as disposing of naturally dying cells. Normally they just perform these tidying-up tasks, until they are summoned to confront new invading microbes. Macrophages arrive first to the scene of many pathogenic assaults. They crawl toward and engulf arriving microbes. These were relatively dormant monocytes in the blood, about two billion circulating at any one time, until vitamin D helps them to mature to be devastating eating machines, when the need arises. At that point, macrophages in turn alert the helper T cells of the adaptive immune system, but we haven't gotten there quite yet.

There are additional chemical signals that alert macrophages to the presence of dangerous infection, taking them to a hyperactive state, enlarging them, and increasing their chemical power to devour pathogens. The most studied of these chemicals are cytokines, particularly a cytokine known as interferon gamma (IFN-gamma) that is produced by another innate immune cell, the natural killer cells. Then macrophages produce another cytokine, tumor necrosis factor, which directly kills cancerous cells and virus-infected cells, and can activate other immune players.

Macrophages need back-up when the body is invaded, and thus dog-whistle their allies the neutrophils by means of interleukin-1 (IL-1), which is a type of cytokine, or chemical signaling system.   A half-hour later, neutrophils are at the site of infection, ready for murderous assault. Neutrophils are so deadly to the pathogens they engulf that they liquefy their prey. There are 20 billion of these vicious killers circulating throughout the body at any time.

In response to the alarm from macrophages, neutrophils that have been speeding along their path in the bloodstream, then – by means of multiple chemical signals – begin to stick to the interior walls of blood vessels, gradually roll to a stop, then pry apart cells of the blood vessel walls, exit the bloodstream, and then go into the infected tissues, where they actively eat pathogens. The feast ensues, where macrophages and neutrophils swallow and destroy invading pathogens.

Vaccines are not yet relevant to this detailed and intensely synergistic immune activity.

Natural killer (NK) cells similarly circulate in the blood until needed at a site of viral infection, and then migrate there, where they kill human cells that have been infected by viruses, bacteria or other pathogens. NK cells also can signal macrophages to hyper-activate and to step up the attack. Through positive feedback, the numbers and potency of each is increased.

Complement is another feature of the innate immune system. These are proteins produced by the liver and abundant in the blood and throughout bodily tissues that are especially lethal to bacteria and other microbes. They are quite poisonous and directly punch holes in or otherwise destroy invaders, but our own cells have so many defenses against complement that we remain unharmed by these naturally produced poisons. Chemical differences between our own cells and invader cells help guide the work of complement to harm the invaders but not to harm us.

Complement can attract and strengthen macrophages, to make their work more potent. Complement places obvious signs on viruses, by attaching signaling molecules to viruses, which notify macrophages and neutrophils to attack them. Complement can also directly destroy viruses.

Interferon is the cytokine mentioned before that human cells produce when viruses are nearby. This chemical interferes with viral entry and replication, and serves as a warning signal to nearby cells to produce it also. The blood cells best equipped to make Type 1 interferon, which is our strongest type of interferon, are dendritic cells. These ingest the pieces and debris of foreign pathogens and carry them to the lymph, where T cells will be developed.

The above may seem to be state-of-the-art high tech design, but the innate immune system has worked this way for millions of years.

Incidentally, nothing involved with a vaccine has shown up yet, except if a prior vaccine happens to significantly match the current attacking pathogen. This has been especially problematic with respiratory viruses, which mutate so quickly that every vaccine used against them has been obsolete by the time of mass distribution, such as flu shots with 14% effectivity, and the COVID vaccines, which do not match the Delta or Omicron or subsequent strains, etc. But that's okay, because most infectious assaults on the body are dealt with by the innate immune system within just a few days, especially with adequate vitamin D available. More on that later.

Cell Count and % of white blood cells per milliliter (ml) of blood, adult human

Innate immune system				Adaptive immune system		
Cell type	% of all white blood cells[299]	Count per ml of blood		Cell type	% of all white blood cells	Count per ml of blood
Neutrophils	53.8%	2,690,000		T-cells	22.5%	1,125,000
Monocytes	8.4%	420,000		B-cells	5.2%	260,000
Natural killer cells	4.4%	220,000				
Eosinophils	3.2%	160,000				
Basophils	1.0%	50,000				
Dendritic cells	1.0%	50,000				
TOTAL INNATE	**71.8%**	**3,590,000**		**TOTAL ADAPTIVE**	**27.7%**	**1,385,000**

There are 5×10^9 = 5 billion red blood cells per milliliter of blood. There are 5×10^6 = 5 million white blood cells per milliliter of blood. Some would argue that red blood cells are also an important component of the innate immune system, because they can produce cytokines and can increase the numbers of and influence activity of other immune cells, such as neutrophils, macrophages and monocytes, and because they carry oxygen to tissues. We have 20 to 25 trillion red blood cells in the body. This is roughly 1,000 times the number of neutrophils and 2,000 or 3,000 times the number of lymphocytes, and it is about 10,000 to 20,000 times the number of B-cells, which are the target cell of vaccine activity.

The adaptive immune system is the smaller part of the human immune system. I say this because lymphocytes are less than 30% (with wide variation in individuals) of the white blood cells in a complete blood count, and less than two-tenths of one percent of all blood cells. B-cells are anywhere from one to twenty percent of all lymphocytes at any given time. This means that probably less than 0.004% (or 4 in 100,000) of all cells in the blood are targeted by vaccines. In the generous scenario that all T-cells are stimulated and boosted by vaccines, that would raise the count to 0.1% (or one in one thousand) of all cells in the blood that would be stimulated by vaccines.

In a brazenly deceptive article published in *Nature*, it is asserted that "functional virus-specific memory CD8 T-cells can be detected in humans for several decades following acute viral infections or immunization with live attenuated vaccines," while the two studies cited in support of this claim did not show anything at all about this occurring following immunization. [300]

There is not any convincing evidence that T-cells are reliably and permanently influenced by vaccination. There have been reported brief dead-cat-bounce effects on T-cells in vitro following vaccines while using heavy laboratory manipulation. Although there have been long-anticipated long-term effects of vaccines on T-cells, it seems the only reliable immune-provoking effect of any vaccines, both the older attenuated and live vaccines up through the mRNA vaccines, is to stimulate B-cell activity, to make antibodies to more quickly attack the exact same invader in the future. But will you ever meet that exact same invader again? SARS-CoV-2 is a RNA virus, and those are notorious for fast change, [301] which is one reason why they have evaded successful vaccine development over the years.

And even if you did meet that exact virus again, knowing what you now know about COVID vaccine risks, would you take that plunge, knowing that only 4 in 100,000 of your blood cells (that is the B cells) might be assisted by the vaccine?
The purpose of a vaccine is to accomplish a task that the innate immune system already does. That is to indicate to the adaptive immune system which pathogens are dangerous and which are not. In the event of a threatening pathogen, whether bacteria, viruses, fungi or parasites, it is the innate immune system that stirs the adaptive immune system to activity, and it is the innate immune system that determines which components – of T cells and / or B cells – will be activated, as challenged and honed by ages of real world training in our ancestors.

The immune system cannot be expected to be self-sufficient, however. Every cell mentioned above in both the innate and adaptive immune systems is stimulated and developed by vitamin D, and cannot function well without it. This then is the most true, broad-spectrum and valuable vaccine, along with moderate amounts of its synergistic partners, the other basic nutrients: vitamins, minerals and amino acids. My book *The Defeat of COVID* cites 130 studies about the immune functions of vitamin D, its effects in strengthening and developing every single type of cell mentioned above and specifically regarding the spectrum of immune effects on SARS-CoV-2 and COVID disease.

Chapter 10

Would you buy a used car from these companies?

People all over the world have been pressured to take Pfizer, Moderna or Johnson & Johnson injections, before being informed of those companies' histories.

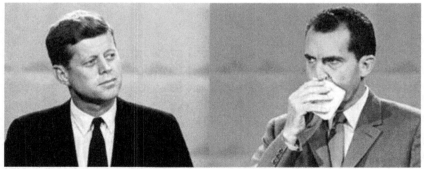

JFK asked Americans: "Would you buy a used car from this man?

Many people already know that in 2009 Pfizer paid the largest criminal fine in US history. This $2.3 billion fine was for healthcare fraud. The Guardian reported the event. [302]

Many people have also learned, after many years of household use, that asbestos was used by Johnson and Johnson in baby powder for decades, an undisclosed toxin in widespread use all over the world. Reuters reported on that. [303]

But what do we know of Moderna, a company that had never previously made a vaccine, nor even a product, as reported by Fortune in 2020? [304]

Igor Chudov wrote about a patented cancer gene from 2017, a 19-nucleotide oncogene sequence, that *somehow* ended up in the SARS-CoV-2 virus, despite a one in a trillion or so odds of that happening just by chance. The patent holder is Moderna. [305] This is that patent. [306]

US009587003B2

(12) **United States Patent**
Bancel et al.

(10) **Patent No.:** US 9,587,003 B2
(45) **Date of Patent:** Mar. 7, 2017

(54) **MODIFIED POLYNUCLEOTIDES FOR THE PRODUCTION OF ONCOLOGY-RELATED PROTEINS AND PEPTIDES**

(71) Applicant: **Moderna Therapeutics, Inc.,** Cambridge, MA (US)

61/618,873, filed on Apr. 2, 2012, provisional application No. 61/681,650, filed on Aug. 10, 2012, provisional application No. 61/737,147, filed on Dec. 14, 2012, provisional application No. 61/618,878, filed on Apr. 2, 2012, provisional application No. 61/681,654, filed on Aug. 10, 2012, provisional

Notice that Stephane Bancel, CEO of Moderna, is listed as the first inventor. At first, I wondered if Chudov could prove what he was writing, and I began to look for the genetic sequence in the fine print of the patent, but there was a lot to sift through, so I set that homework aside. Then, astonishingly, Bancel himself admitted to FOX Business that yes, this very event was possible. [307]

Here are my questions:

1) As a naturopathic oncologist, I have worked with cancer patients for the last 15 years. All that time, I have used time-honored natural ingredients in IV nutrients, the ones we have known for many decades:

vitamin C, B vitamins, minerals, and I explain how they work at length to patients and the public, both in my books and online. If I had done what Moderna did, if I came anywhere near – within miles of – inventing a pro-cancer gene, and then actually having the nerve to patent such a thing, do you think any cancer patient would come within miles of me ever again? And then if I had it inserted into a known bio-weapon in a bio-weapon lab, would any sane person come anywhere near even one item that I produced? Would anyone buy so much as a used car from me? Cancer patients actually want to fight cancer, not visit with a pro-cancer poison maker. And not just a pro-cancer poison maker who would inject lab mice with such nastiness, but rather disperse it into the human population via an engineered coronavirus? If I were then brazen enough to invent a vaccine, would any sane or well-informed person trust me so much with that very first vaccine, that they would actually irreversibly inject such a wacko concoction?

2) Considering Pfizer's $2.3 billion record-setting felony fine was for drug fraud, would any sane or knowledgeable person consider taking any drug that Pfizer made ever again? Much less an irreversible injection, where the ingredients have not been fully disclosed?

3) Considering that everyone knows how very deadly asbestos is, and its connection with mesothelioma, would any sane or self-respecting person take a product made by a company that hid asbestos in an over-the-counter product for decades?

Well, so much for the COVID vaccines, which we know have negative efficacy and a horrific pattern of deaths and injuries, as I write about in the first five chapters of this book.

For COVID prevention and treatment, that only leaves the early treatments that have been working successfully all over the world, such as in the meta-analyses and randomized controlled trials on nearly all continents. The most comprehensive information that I have seen on that is here: https://c19early.com/ My book *The Defeat Of COVID* explains how the best-performing and safest early treatments, vitamin D, zinc, hydroxychloroquine and ivermectin, work against COVID or any viral respiratory infection, and data showing how masks, lockdowns, testing and vaccines have not worked. [308]

Fortunately, more of the world is starting to imagine a future without the COVID vaccines. Doses of manufactured COVID vaccines will soon arrive to their expiration dates. Statens Serum Institut, an agency of the Danish government, has found that the global supply of vaccines exceeds the demand, and " . . .in light of declining demand . . . it has been difficult for Denmark and other EU countries to find recipient countries for excess doses." [309] Similarly, the uptake of booster shots is considerably lower than for the earlier doses of COVID vaccines.

Alternatives to vaccination for COVID

Chapter 11

Vitamin D beats the vaccines against COVID

Vaccines only work on adaptive, not innate, immunity. Vitamin D does a much better job with both.

Adaptive immunity and the COVID vaccines

The adaptive immune system comprises T-cells and B-cells (lymphocytes), and it is the smaller part of the human immune system. I say this because T-cells and B-cells are less than 30% (with wide variation in individuals) of the white blood cells in a complete blood count, and are less than two tenths of one percent (0.2%) of all blood cells. B-cells, which are the cells on which vaccines act, are anywhere from one to twenty percent of all lymphocytes at any given time. This means that probably less than 0.004% (or 4 in 100,000) of all cells in the blood are targeted by vaccines and can produce antibodies. In the generous (but highly unlikely) scenario that all T-cells might be stimulated and boosted by vaccines, that would raise the count to 0.1% (or one in one thousand) of all cells in the blood that would be stimulated by vaccines.

Vaccine manufacturers have focused, as they must in every vaccine for it to address advertised claims, on recognizable proteins produced by a pathogen. In the case of COVID, that protein is a spike protein. A second encounter with a pathogenic microbe, following either naturally acquired infection or the vaccine, arouses immunological memory. That subsequent encounter with a pathogen is a larger and faster response than in the first encounter. Often these are so fast and forceful that an individual can clear a virus before even being aware of its presence. This is an asymptomatic defeat of the virus. The goal of vaccination is for the vaccinated individual to experience no disease from the pathogen.

There are enormous and mounting problems with the use of vaccines against COVID. One of the earliest known problems is that vaccines against coronaviruses have never worked. [310] Other early problems with the COVID vaccines used in 2021 (from late 2020) include their hasty development and lack of animal trials, and lack of informed consent, and political and financial pressure to take vaccines. mRNA vaccines have had animal [311] and human trials, which failed abysmally. [312] The COVID vaccines were likely doomed to fail because they combined several known red flags for disaster: mRNA, lipid nano-particles (highly inflammatory), Polyethylene glycol (PEG) (known to be highly and dangerously allergenic), and addressing a coronavirus. All of these four factors had been known to scientists in various fields to be very problematic already.

Then, compounding this growing catastrophe with the COVID vaccines, professor of viral immunology Byram Bridle discusses how corners were cut, the phase three clinical trials were skipped, which forced the public on which the vaccines were used to become the phase three clinical trial subjects, of course, unbeknownst to them: "Those being vaccinated now are, whether they realize it or not, part of the phase three experiment." [313] This is aside from the enormous problems now being learned regarding the lack of safety and lack of efficacy, in fact negative efficacy of these vaccines. [314]

For those of you who have not submitted to these vaccines, and even for those who have, I would suggest being very glad that vitamin D exists and is widely available. This chapter will examine effects of vitamin D, achieving far more protection of the human body in the adaptive immune realm than vaccines can even begin to achieve, and this has been amply demonstrated with regard to SARS-CoV-2 and COVID.

Adaptive immunity and Vitamin D

Vitamin D receptors have been found in abundance in activated lymphocytes. [315] [316] Whereas multiple lymphocytes contain vitamin D receptors, CD-8 lymphocytes, also known as cytotoxic T-cells, were found to have the highest concentration, and vitamin D was found to increase the number of those receptors. [317] However, vitamin D also regulates helper T cells, notably TH1, TH2 and TH17, as well as the regulatory T cells that play an essential role in the prevention of auto-immune disease. Where vitamin D is deficient, T-lymphocytes are shown to be pathogenic. [318]

TH1 helper T cells tend to be more pro-inflammatory; their cytokines include interleukin-2 (IL-2), interferon gamma (IFN-gamma) and tumor necrosis factor (TNF)-alpha. Vitamin D tends to suppress TH1, switching adaptive immune response to TH2. [319] For example, the vitamin D receptor (VDR) inhibits the T-cell cytokine IL-2. [320] In contrast, vitamin D tends to enhance TH2 helper T-cell proliferation and cytokine production. TH2 T-cells are more anti-inflammatory and those cells excrete such cytokines as the interleukins IL-3, IL-4, IL-5 and IL-10. [321] [322]

Vitamin D3 has shown association with priming naïve human T cells, specifically CD4 and CD8 T lymphocytes, to enhance their migration to sites of infection.[323] The expression and activity of vitamin D receptors are important for every stage examined in the life of a T-lymphocyte, including development, differentiation and expression of effector functions.[324]

Vitamin D vs viral infections

In the presence of pathogenic respiratory viruses, normal lung epithelial cells convert 25-hydroxy vitamin D (which is the inactive or storage form of vitamin D) to the active form, namely 1,25-hydroxyvitamin D3, which is the active form.[325] Cathelicidins are stimulated by vitamin D, and are essential to defense against viruses. Vitamin D also stimulates the powerful Type I Interferons (IFNs) which in turn stimulate expression of over 100 IFN-stimulated genes, which show a variety of antiviral activities.[326] [327] Vitamin D also showed evidence of inhibiting viral replication.[328]

COVID has been compared to respiratory syncytial virus (RSV) in that both have shown life-threatening amounts of inflammatory chemokines in the airways. In both diseases, this process has been a part of its pathogenesis, severity of the infection and mortality.[329] Modest improvement in each is obtainable with prescribed corticosteroids,[330] but vitamin D gave more consistent response in RSV treatment.[331] Even the intractable human immunodeficiency virus (HIV-1) has shown susceptibility to vitamin D treatment.[332] [333]

Significantly improved outcomes of respiratory infections have been seen with vitamin D supplementation and / or higher serum levels, in terms of shorter hospitalization, lower cost of care and lower mortality. [334] [335] In a study of 18,883 individuals, there was an increased prevalence of upper respiratory tract infection in those having less than 30 ng/ml serum levels of 25-hydroxy vitamin D compared to those having 30 ng/ml and above. This association was even stronger than season, body mass index, history of asthma or smoking or chronic obstructive pulmonary disease (COPD). [336] Pneumonia patients with < 12 ng/ml 25-hydroxy vitamin D levels had higher mortality at 30 days. [337] Children also showed correlation between low vitamin D levels and pneumonia and acute lower respiratory infection. [338] [339] Likewise, vitamin D deficiency in children was associated with more likelihood of hospitalization, severity of disease and longer hospitalization for respiratory infections. [340]

This chapter is part of a series on Vitamin D, with regard to its effects against SARS-CoV-2 in particular and viral infections in general, and the successfully life-saving results that vitamin D has shown against SARS-CoV-2, COVID and its variants. That series is on https://colleenhuber.substack.com.

Avoiding the COVID Vaccines

Chapter 12

Religious exemption language

When human rights abuses are inflicted against workers' constitutional rights, there are legal ways to resist.

What happened to the Biden Administration's OSHA "mandate" in the US Supreme Court?

Five Supreme Court justices, in this January 2022 case, acted in a way (except for a thin thread of possible excuse, as I discuss below) that possibly violated the Constitution and federal law. Except that they did not create a new mandate; they simply stayed an existing one not of their creation, and they kicked the matter back to lower courts to be decided in more detailed litigation there. However, by that time, healthcare workers, those with legal standing, will have been irreversibly injected in gross violation of every contemporary understanding of human rights.

I am referring to the Center for Medicare and Medicaid Services (CMS) mandate forcing healthcare workers whose employers receive Medicare / Medicaid funds to be injected with COVID vaccines, whether they want to or not. Notably all four dissenting justices, Thomas, Alito, Gorsuch and Barrett, wrote dissenting opinions. In a 5-4 vote, the majority ruled to allow Biden's mandate that healthcare workers in Medicare / Medicaid facilities must be forced to take the COVID vaccines, or lose their jobs. In doing so, the five justices in the majority ignored the following laws and international treaties.

- the Tenth Amendment to the US Constitution, which defers any powers to the states or to the people that are not delegated to the federal government by the Constitution. I am not an attorney, but I am quite sure that neither the US government nor state or local governments has ever been granted authority to medicate (or to inject or to force inject or to force medicate) any citizen, regardless of type of work.

- Arguably the First Amendment, protecting freedom of religion and freedom of speech, considering that action (i.e., refusing a vaccine) is an expressive act, and has been previously considered as a form of speech.

- The Fourteenth Amendment provides for equal protection under the laws. It would be a flagrant violation to force a healthcare worker to be subject to unwanted medical treatment when fellow citizens are not.

- Practicing medicine without a license: I have been told by an attorney that this is a violation of criminal law in all 50 states. I am not an attorney and cannot speak about that knowledgeably. But I would think that even Supreme Court justices may not prescribe a medical treatment without a license to practice medicine.

- Practicing forced medicine on those who do not want it. This is the biggest elephant in the room. This is a violation of federal informed consent law 45 CFR §46.116 and much of the rest of 45 CFR §46, as the only COVID vaccines available in the US to date are experimental and under "Emergency Use Authorization." (Comirnaty was FDA approved, but is not yet available anywhere in the US, nor will be this year, we are told.) Practicing forced medicine also violates the Nuremberg Code and the Universal Declaration of Human Rights and the Helsinki Declaration. Some of history's most noxious barbarians chose to administer some form of poisons to their victims. Information already gathered by the US federal government, Department of Health and Human Services' own database, VAERS, showed that the COVID vaccines have caused more deaths in only one year than all other vaccines combined over the last 30 years. [341] [342] I explain more specifically in Chapter 6 how that happened:

The Nuremberg Code arose out of humanity's essential need to prevent another Holocaust. Attorney Mary Holland says, "If we learned anything from World War II, it's that medical procedures must not be forced on individuals." I think she means even medical procedures that could very well turn out to be benign, and that your well-meaning relatives and co-workers urge you to get.

The bottom line from a human rights perspective is:

Your medicine may be my poison, and I alone decide that.

Even without the Supreme Court decision, is there any obligation to comply with an unconstitutional law? From Marbury vs Madison 5 US 137: Any law, mandate or other that is "repugnant to the Constitution is null and void."

Understanding the fundamental principles of human rights enshrined in the US Constitution and the Nuremberg Code should have been a strict requirement for all of these justices at various checkpoints in their development as middle school and high school graduates, let alone as attorneys and then jurists. Every doctor and pharmacist knows this principle well: Never force, coerce, threaten or even unduly pressure a medical treatment on a patient. As a physician, I was required to study informed consent principles in medical jurisprudence courses both in medical school and later in my role as an IRB member. That later training was done in seminars given by the Office of Human Research Protections of the US Department of Health and Human Services (HHS). How were these justices exempt from such basic human rights and federal informed consent law training? How was Biden exempt?

Justice Clarence Thomas understands the issue well. In his dissent, Justice Thomas wrote, "These cases are not about the efficacy or importance of COVID-19 vaccines. They are only about whether CMS has the statutory authority to force healthcare workers, by coercing their employers, to undergo a medical procedure they do not want and cannot undo." [343]

But here we are, amid the shambles of the Schwab / Gates concocted great reset / digital passport / 'we own you and your possessions' reset, which by the way suffered an important defeat in that January 2022 Supreme Court case, because the great news of that day was that the OSHA mandate was rejected by the Supreme Court. Now most Americans are not likely to be inflicted with a digital vaccine passport-enabled China-type social credit system, at least any time soon. Or at least, the resetters will have some considerable hurdles before they could push the US to that point, after the Supreme Court's OSHA ruling.

But SCOTUS did rubber stamp on that day the (what I believe to be) clearly unconstitutional and illegal assault on the bodily autonomy, personal choice and medical wisdom of medical professionals.

Many healthcare workers have been too intimidated by threats of job loss to openly resist the new biofascists, but have fought back with various non-compliance, passive resistance, contractual demands (such as you, employer, must agree in writing to un-inject your witches' brew from me before I leave work each day), and other perfectly legitimate forms of civil disobedience, disrespect and inconvenient obstacles against their knuckle-dragging employers who opted for a human rights-violated, vaccine-sickened and resentful workforce. Heckuva job, bosses!

Religious exemption and medical exemption

Even in this debacle of human rights abuse from the majority decision, there is a window of hope left open by the Supreme Court's ruling of January 2022: Religious exemption and medical exemption. In the Court's opinion on the CMS case:

"The Secretary of Health and Human Services administers the Medicare and Medicaid programs, which provide health insurance for millions of elderly, disabled, and low income Americans. In November 2021, the Secretary announced that, in order to receive Medicare and Medicaid funding, participating facilities must ensure that their staff—***unless exempt for medical or religious reasons***—are vaccinated against COVID–19. 86 Fed. Reg. 61555 (2021). Two District Courts enjoined enforcement of the rule, and the Government now asks us to stay those injunctions. Agreeing that it is entitled to such relief, we grant the applications." [Emphasis mine]. [344]

Religious exemption requires no outside stamp of approval, such as from a physician, as it is a declaration by an individual. Although some have argued that an employer may deny such an exemption (the Interim Rule), the US government itself confirms that "Title VII of the Civil Rights Act of 1964 prohibits employers from discriminating against individuals because of their religion (or lack of religious belief) in hiring, firing, or any other terms and conditions of employment." And: "It is also unlawful to retaliate against an individual for opposing employment practices that discriminate based on religion . . . " [345]

I am not an attorney, but I can opine that the Civil Rights Act seems to be prohibitive against an employer's attempt to deny religious exemption. The Supreme Court has previously honored any "sincerely held religious belief" as adequate ground for religious exemption. The Religious Freedom Restoration Act [346] reinforces the First Amendment and was upheld earlier this month, even in defense of the First Amendment rights of military service members. Religious exemption is a declaration made by an individual, backed by the First Amendment and now acknowledged again in this January 2022 Supreme Court ruling.

Here is some language used with employers that has been seen to be successful in the COVID era for expressing religious objection, and thus asserting religious exemption to the COVID vaccines. How do I already know this, when the SCOTUS decision came down only recently? Because here in Arizona we have long had some of the strongest exemptions to vaccines of any states, including religious exemption. And that fact is exactly what brought my family here decades ago. Now 100,000s of families have made the same or similar exodus to the free states. In Arizona, we see this especially from California, skyrocketing our housing prices, but that's another topic.

Already several dozen patients of mine (including MDs, RNs, pharmacists, pilots and flight attendants, but even more, workers in large companies) have kept their jobs in the COVID era using some variation of some of the following language for religious exemption from vaccines.

If you agree, and especially if you feel strong agreement with any of the following, (I am not an attorney, so cannot say confidently, but would think that) it would rise to the level of sincerely held religious belief:

- 1 Corinthians 6:19 - "The body is the temple of the spirit." A logical corollary to this is not to recklessly trash the body with experimental treatments, especially substances that have already proven to be toxic.

- COVID vaccines were developed using tissue cloned from aborted fetal cells. I do not support that industry, and do not want that cannibalistic abomination injected into me.

- A Harvard study has shown that exogenous mRNA can change DNA. [347] If I am forced to risk changing my DNA, am I still the creature that God created? Or do I then become somebody's genetic experiment?

- The right to bodily autonomy is inherent in each human being and is God-given. I am not a member of any religion that condones forced injection of anything, even saline, into the body of an unwilling person.

- My refusal to participate in the vaccine superstition cult is my expression of my sincerely held religious belief.

Each of the above statements have been made by multiple people known to me to have been used successfully with their employers. Recently, COVID era topics are the topics that my patients want to discuss most avidly, so I get a lot of information from them about what has worked with their and their family members' employers.

If you think some of the above language would be useful to a healthcare worker or to a resident of one of the cities that have fallen to biofascism, such as NYC, Chicago, etc, please share it with them.

"Stand therefore, having your loins girt about with truth, ... ye shall be able to quench all the fiery darts of the wicked."

- Ephesians 6:14-16

Chapter 13

Medical Exemption

Zyklon B was forced on unwilling people in the 1940's. The COVID vaccines were forced on unwilling people last year. But not on my watch. Here's why.

Of the thousands of patient appointments I've had in the COVID era, I've often been in the role of patient advocate, but with a particular urgency in working with people who found themselves coerced by their employers to submit to COVID vaccines. (Such coercion is in clear violation of federal law, [348] as the reader likely knows.) Medical doctors, nurses, other hospital workers, pharmacists, flight attendants, pilots, and especially those working for companies of more than 100 employees have come to me for medical exemption from vaccines.

Of those, I found the pharmacists to be the most memorable demographic, for three reasons:

First, pharmacists (PharmD) are the most specifically educated in drug toxicity of any class of professional. That pharmacists would have to come to a naturopathic physician to receive a medical exemption from a forced injection, one which is known by them to be poisonous, would have been unimaginable until 2021.

I'll never forget what a pharmacist told me in one of these visits: "The most important principle I learned in my PharmD education was to never force a medication on a patient. So why is my employer forcing this on me?"

Then there were other stories, from people who knew pharmacists who would no longer be willing to administer the covid vaccines, whether refusing to take appointments for those, or who outright quit retail pharmacy altogether, leaving pharmacies so short-staffed that many have closed. [349] People who had never had an issue with timely pickup of their non-controversial blood pressure medications of a decade's use now sometimes find it difficult getting even these filled on time. [350]

The covid vaccines have not been so fondly received by pharmacy staff as the powers-that-be had assumed. There are grapevine stories of people who know from others of multiple full vaccine vials going into the trash routinely last year, and suspected tremendous numbers of saline or other harmless shots and nothing shots of needle only, instead of the clotshot. I have heard of this compassion being directed especially to frail seniors, teens railroaded by vaccine cult parents, and people who confided to the pharmacist, "I don't want this, but my job is making me." However, there are pharmacists who now flat out refuse to give COVID vaccines to anyone, especially recently, since all the revelations of harm.

I think it's fair to say that the CDC boast of 77.4% of Americans partially or fully vaccinated [351] is almost as crazily false as their claims of "safe and effective." Having an ear to the ground in the Phoenix area, with especially keen interest in this issue over the last year, and from a number of different industries' employees, including hospital, insurance, pharmacy and transportation, including among local and nationwide management, all speaking confidentially to me, and all without direct knowledge of the same, the actual number of COVID-vaccinated is likely between 45% and 50%, minus those who have since died from the vaccines.

I write medical exemptions for all who ask, because it is a fundamental principle of medical ethics, and what mainly separates us from fascists, that nobody should be subjected to a medical treatment that they do not want. Together with the Hippocratic Oath, First Do No Harm, these are the two most important principles in medicine. So my medical exemptions all read the same, as follows:

"Medically exempt from ALL COVID vaccines, due to known and proven risks of severe injury."

There is no need, nor justification, to violate a patient's privacy to their employers by saying the vaccine can't be taken due to heart disease or family history of heart disease or other condition or vulnerability to the same. Rather, the fact that the COVID vaccines are known to be poisonous is enough of a reason for a medical exemption, and the fact that the person does not want it is way more of a good reason, a decisive and pinnacle jurisdiction reason, not to have it. I am not an attorney. By "pinnacle jurisdiction" reason, I mean that the patient has the final and ultimately decisive say regarding what goes into his or her body, including any medical treatments to be taken. I am not interested in government or media pronouncements to the contrary. The sovereignty of the human body is non-negotiable in a post-slavery society, and our rights are inalienable. I know that one of my exemptions was rejected by a Colorado employer and one by a local employer, but in both cases, religious exemption was then used successfully.

States such as California have made it clear that anyone who does what I do should not have a license to practice medicine, and Toby Rogers PhD describes the California law as "the most draconian anti-science law [he has] ever seen." [352]

If such fascist laws as California's SB 276 and SB 277 ever took hold in Arizona, there would be fierce court battles. If I were involved, there would be a merciless barrage of data and court-ordered Pfizer documents [353] that I would submit to the court(s) to defend my medical exemption(s), and more importantly, my patients' right to have it. I have submitted to other courts testimony that is contained in Chapter 2 of this book, regarding the now known negative efficacy and the alarming risks of the COVID vaccines. The 1/11/22 draft of that material quickly became out-of-date, as additional damning evidence against these vaccines is now in the public domain since I wrote it, and I have updated that for Chapter 2 in this book.

If the powers-that-be want to stop me from writing medical exemptions from poisonous products, they've got a hellcat legal fight on their hands.

"Find out what people will submit to,
and you have found out
the exact amount of injustice and wrong
which will be imposed on them."

- Frederick Douglass

Chapter 14

Medical Freedom in US Courts: Court Cases That Have Upheld Bodily Autonomy

The right to refuse medical treatment has a long history of judicial recognition in US state and federal courts. This list of cases that are pertinent to bodily autonomy shows the link to each case with quotes from each ruling judge.

Introduction

The history of legal torts has long recognized the physical security of one's body. It is referred to in the 39th Article of the *Magna Carta*. The English jurist Sir William Blackstone, writing in 1753, identified "the right of personal security" to include life, limb, health and reputation. [354] He identified personal security as one of the three elements of "liberty," with the other two elements being personal liberty and private property.

The history of US judicial recognition of medical freedom has often hinged on individuals' right to refuse unwanted medical intervention, whether examination or testing or treatments.

There are two strong legal bases for upholding this right of refusal. First, the US Constitution guarantees privacy, which prohibits governmental intrusion on medical decision-making by the individual. The reader will note that the cases below cite the 1st, 3rd, 4th, 5th, 8th, 9th and 14th Amendments, although it seems the 13th Amendment may be equally applicable, because if a human must not be owned or enslaved or conscripted to involuntary servitude by others, then logically that person's body and bodily decisions must not be controlled by others. Also, common law guarantees individuals the right to informed consent for any medical interaction, along with its corollary, the right of refusal to consent to any proposed medical treatment, without coercion, harassment or punishment.

The preponderance of judicial rulings on the right to refuse medical treatment have upheld this right of refusal, and so strongly that the reader will find below that courts have prohibited doctors, hospitals and government actors from violating it. It has been clear throughout US history, and in the cases listed below, that mentally competent adults, and even many with diagnosed mental illness, as well as prisoners and "mature minors," have the right to refuse medical treatment, even if that treatment may be life-saving, and even if that treatment may be disapproved of by the medical profession or others.

Ronald B Standler compiled a list of judicial decisions throughout US history that pertain to individuals' right to refuse medical treatment. His essay on this topic covers about 80 cases. [355] This more abridged summary of some of those court cases, as well as several more, contains accessible links to settled court cases in the US.

The following compilation aims to provide more extensive quotations from the justices' opinions when pertinent to the right to refuse medical treatment and its historical support in the courts, with specific attention to court rulings on individuals' rights to refuse medical interactions, exams, procedures and treatments.

This topic also is involved with the right to privacy and bodily autonomy and informed consent. The judges cite the US Constitution and its Amendments as well as statutory law.

Disclaimers

1) I am not an attorney, and even if I were, I would not and do not offer general legal advice. Clearly a qualified attorney in one's own state or in the state with jurisdiction where a dispute arises would be an appropriate expert to consult regarding a dispute or action or legal advice. I am a physician of 15 years and medical expert witness in court cases that are somewhat similar to these cases, but I do not share my opinion on any of the cases listed below, with one exception: the highly anomalous Jacobson vs Massachusetts case of 1905, discussed at the end of the article, as well as the Introduction section at the beginning of this article. The quotes shown below are all from the judges' rulings in the respective cases.

2) Judicial opinions are attributed to the judges who authored them, and no other person holds the copyright to those, and I quote them only with attribution to the court opinions.

United States federal and state court cases pertaining to the right to refuse medical procedures, informed consent, and bodily autonomy

1891: Union Pacific Railway Co vs Botsford, 141 US 250, 251.

https://www.law.cornell.edu/supremecourt/text/141/250

In this landmark case, considered to be one of the most important for bodily autonomy, Justice Gray referred to the "inviolability of the person," and cited prior references to it in our constitutional history.

After an injury, the railway demanded medical examination of Botsford, who refused. The court upheld Botsford's right not to be examined, and stated:

"No right is held more sacred or more carefully guarded by the common law, than the right of every individual to the possession and control of his own person, free from all restraint or interference of others, unless by clear and unquestionable authority of law."

"The right to one's person may be said to be a right of complete immunity; to be let alone."

1914: Schloendorff vs Society of New York Hospital, 105 NE 92, 93 New York

https://biotech.law.lsu.edu/cases/consent/schoendorff.htm

"In the case at hand, the wrong complained of is not merely negligence. It is trespass. Every human being of adult years and sound mind has a right to determine what shall be done with his own body; and a surgeon who performs an operation without his patient's consent commits an assault, for which he is liable in damages."

"The fact that the wrong complained of here is trespass rather than negligence, distinguishes this case from most of the cases that have preceded it."

1958: England vs Louisiana State Board of Medical Examiners. 259 F 2d. 626, 627. 5th Circuit. 1959: Cert. denied. 359 US 1012.

https://casetext.com/case/england-v-louisiana-state-board-of-med-exam

" . . . the State cannot deny to any individual the right to exercise a reasonable choice in the method of treatment of his ills, . . . "

1962: Erickson vs Dilgard. 252 New York 2d. 705, 706. New York Superior Court.

https://casetext.com/case/matter-of-erickson-v-dilgard

In the matter of an adult with internal bleeding who refused a blood transfusion, the Court ruled: "It is the individual who is the subject of a medical decision who has the final say and that this must necessarily be so in a system of government which gives the greatest possible protection to the individual in the furtherance of his own desires."

1965: In re Brooks' Estate. 205 NE 2d 435. Illinois.

https://www.casemine.com/judgement/us/5914c89eadd7b049347ebd5c

Brooks had refused blood transfusion on both religious and medical grounds, but received transfusions despite her expressed wishes.

"It is established that the commands of the First Amendment to the United States Constitution relating to religious freedom are embraced within the Fourteenth Amendment and by it extended to the States." Cantwell vs Connecticut, 310 US 296, 303, 84. L.ed. 1213, 60 S.CT 900, 903. School District of Abington Township vs Schempp, 374 US 203, 215, 10. L.ed.2d 844, 83 S CT. 1560, 1568.

"The controversy [of conformity vs nonconformity to religious beliefs] culminated in the First Amendment's guarantee to the individual of freedom from governmental domination in his religious beliefs and practices. . . ." Reynolds vs United States, 98 US 145, 25. L.ed. 244. Davis vs Beason, 133 US 333, 33 L.ed. 637.

"In the final analysis, what has happened here involves a judicial attempt to decide what course of action is best for a particular individual, notwithstanding that indivdual's contrary views based upon religious convictions. Such actions cannot be constitutionally countenanced."

1965: Griswold vs Connecticut. 381 US 479,

https://supreme.justia.com/cases/federal/us/381/479/

The right of privacy is implicit throughout the Bill of Rights.
"A right to privacy can be inferred from several amendments in the Bill of Rights."

1971: Winters vs Miller. 446 F 2d 65. 2d Circuit, US Court of Appeals.

https://casetext.com/case/winters-v-miller

The Court upheld the right to refuse medical treatment.
"It is clear and appellees concede that if we were dealing here with an ordinary patient suffering from a physical ailment, the hospital authorities would have no right to impose compulsory medical treatment against the patient's will and indeed, that to do so would constitute a common law assault and battery. The question then becomes at what point, if at all, does the patient suffering from a mental illness lose the rights he would otherwise enjoy in this regard."

1972: Holmes vs Silver Cross Hospital of Joliet, IL. 340 F Supp. 125, 130. Northern District of Illinois.

https://casetext.com/case/holmes-v-silver-cross-hospital-of-joliet-illinois

"A state-appointed conservator's ordering of medical treatment for a person in violation of his religious beliefs, no matter how well intentioned the conservator may be, violates the First Amendment's freedom of exercise clause in the absence of some substantial state interest."

1972: Canterbury vs Spence. 464 F 2d 772, 780. Washington DC Circuit.

https://biotech.law.lsu.edu/cases/consent/canterbury_v_s pence.htm

"The root premise is the concept, fundamental in American jurisprudence, that 'every human being of adult years and sound mind has a right to determine what shall be done with his own body . . . ' [citing Schloendorff vs Society of New York Hospital, 105 NE 92, 93. New York 1914.]" Cert denied. 409 US 1064, 1972.

"True consent to what happens to one's self is the informed exercise of a choice, and that entails an opportunity to evaluate knowledgeably the options available and the risks attendant upon each."

1972: In re Osborne, 294 A 2d 372 Washington DC.

https://casetext.com/case/in-re-osborne-35

Although a man who was injured by a tree falling on him had two young children, his right to refuse blood transfusion was upheld by the court, beginning with a bedside hearing.

"Judge Bacon took note of a possible overriding state interest based on the fact that the patient had two young children. It was concluded, however, that the maturity of this lucid patient, his long-standing beliefs and those of his family did not justify state intervention."

Associate Judge Yeagley concurred: "Although I concur in the court's opinion, I would add that the thrust of the opinion in my view, while based on the First Amendment, is not . . . based solely on religious freedom, but also on the broader based freedom of choice whether founded on religious beliefs or otherwise."

1972: Cobbs vs Grant. 8 Cal 3d 229, 502 P.2d 1, 104 California Reporter 505.

https://biotech.law.lsu.edu/cases/consent/Cobbs_v_Grant.htm

"A person of adult years and in sound mind has the right, in the exercise of control over his own body, to determine whether or not to submit to lawful medical treatment."

" . . . it is the prerogative of the patient, not the physician, to determine for himself the direction in which he believes his interests lie. To enable the patient to chart his course knowledgeably, reasonable familiarity with the therapeutic alternatives and their hazards becomes essential."

1973: In re Yetter, 62 Pennsylvania D&C 2d 619. Com Pl.

https://cite.case.law/pa-d-c2d/62/619/

Although a 60-year old woman had been found to be schizophrenic and delusional and committed to a state hospital, she was found to be mentally competent to refuse surgery for breast cancer. The patient stated that she was afraid because of the death of her aunt following such surgery, and that it was her own body and she did not desire the operation.

"It is clear that mere commitment to a State hospital for treatment of mental illness does not destroy a person's competency or require the appointment of a guardian of the estate or person.

"In our opinion, the constitutional right of privacy includes the right of a mature competent adult to refuse to accept medical recommendations that may prolong one's life and which, to a third person at least, appear to be in his best interests; in short, that the right of privacy includes a right to die with which the State should not interfere where there are no minor or unborn children and no clear and present danger to public health, welfare or morals. If the person was competent while being presented with the decision and in making the decision which she did, the court should not interfere even though her decision might be considered unwise, foolish or ridiculous."

1976: Matter of Quinlan. 355 A 2d. 647. New Jersey

https://law.justia.com/cases/new-jersey/supreme-court/1976/70-n-j-10-0.html

This well-publicized case considered for the first time whether a patient in a persistent vegetative state could have life support withdrawn. The case upheld the right to refuse medical care to also belong to unconscious patients.

1977: Superintendent of Belchertown State Sch vs Saikewicz 373 Massachusetts 728.

https://law.justia.com/cases/massachusetts/supreme-court/1977/373-mass-728-2.html

"The constitutional right to privacy, as we conceive it, is an expression of the sanctity of individual free choice and self-determination as fundamental constituents of life. The value of life as so perceived is lessened not by a decision to refuse treatment, but by the failure to allow a competent human being the right of choice."

1978: Matter of Quackenbush. 383 A 2d. 785. New Jersey, Morris County.

https://law.justia.com/cases/new-jersey/appellate-division-published/1978/156-n-j-super-282-0.html

A 72 year-old man had gangrene in both legs. Surgery was offered as a way to remove the infection, which the patient refused.

"Always present is the predominant interest in the preservation of life. But constitutional and decision law invest Quackenbush with rights that overcome that interest. Quackenbush, therefore, as a mentally competent individual, has the right to make his informed choice concerning the operation, and I will not interfere with that choice."

1978: Lane vs Candura. 376 NE 2d. 1232, 1236. Massachusetts Appellate Court.

https://law.justia.com/cases/massachusetts/court-of-appeals/1978/6-mass-app-ct-377-1.html

Even if amputation of a gangrenous leg were necessary to save a patient's life, the Court ruled: "The law protects her right to make her own decision to accept or reject treatment, whether that decision is wise or unwise. . . . Mrs. Candura's decision may be regarded by most as unfortunate, but on the record in this case it is not the uninformed decision of a person incapable of appreciating the nature and consequences of her act. We cannot anticipate whether she will reconsider and will consent to the operation, but we are all of the opinion that the operation may not be forced on her against her will."

1978: Satz vs Perlmutter. 362 So 2d 160. Florida Appellate Court.

https://casetext.com/case/satz-v-perlmutter

"It is our conclusion, therefore, under the facts before us, that when these several public policy interests are weighed against the rights of Mr. Perlmutter, the latter must and should prevail. . . . Such a course of conduct [violation of Perlmutter's will] invades the patient's constitutional right of privacy, removes his freedom of choice and invades his right to self-determine."

1980: Andrews vs Ballard. 498 F Supp. 1038 1049. Southern District Texas.

https://law.justia.com/cases/federal/district-courts/FSupp/498/1038/1652028/

At the time of this case, Texas state law and Rules of the Texas State Board of Medical Examiners only allowed licensed physicians to practice acupuncture in the State of Texas. The plaintiffs, 46 residents of Harris County Texas, had sought acupuncture treatment. They argued that the constitutional right of privacy, protected by the Due Process Clause of the Fourteenth Amendment, encompasses the decision to obtain or reject medical treatment and that existing laws impermissibly deprived them of that right because they (a) virtually eliminate the practice of acupuncture in Texas, and (b) are not necessary to serve the State's interest in protecting the health and safety of the patient.

"For the reasons stated herein, it finds that the challenged articles and rules do not withstand constitutional scrutiny."

The Court referred to the right to refuse medical treatment as a privacy right and cited 10 cases, including Union Pacific R Co vs Botsford:

"No right is held more sacred, or is more carefully guarded, by the common law, than the right of every individual to the possession and control of his own person, free from all restraint or interference of others, unless by clear and unquestionable authority of law. As well said by Judge Cooley: 'The right to one's person may be said to be a right of complete immunity; to be let alone.' "

"Since that time, the importance of this right remains unchallenged and undiminished."

1980: Davis vs Hubbard. 506 F Supp. 915, 930-932. Northern District Ohio.

https://law.justia.com/cases/federal/district-courts/FSupp/506/915/1653591/

" . . . this Court notes at the outset its essential agreement with respect to both the existence of the right [to refuse medical treatment] and the factors which determine its shape. But unlike some of the courts which have derived the right to refuse treatment from the First Amendment, the Eighth Amendment, as well as the 'penumbras' and 'shadows' of these and the Third, Fourth, and Fifth Amendments, this Court believes the source of the right can best be understood as substantive due process, or phrased differently, as an aspect of liberty guaranteed by the due process clause of the Fourteenth Amendment."

"Our own constitutional history contains many references to the importance of the 'inviolability of the person.' "

"More specifically, a respect for bodily integrity, 'as the major locus of separation between the individual and the world,' (L Tribe, *American Constitutional Law*) underlies the specific constitutional guarantees of the Fourth Amendment, [4 cases cited], the Eighth Amendment [3 cases cited], as well as the due process clauses of the Fifth and Fourteenth Amendments. [2 cases cited] "

"Closely related to a person's interest in his body is his interest in making decisions about his body. In the law of torts, this interest is reflected in the concept of consent. For example, in the context of medical treatment, treatment by a physician in a non-emergency that is rendered without the patient's informed consent, or exceeds the consent given, is actionable as a battery. See, e.g. Mohr vs Wiliams, 95 932 Minnesota 261, 104 NW 12 (1905); Pratt vs Davis, 224 Illinois 300 79 NE 562 (1906); Rolater vs Strain, 39 Oklahoma 572, 137 P96 (1913); Schloendorff vs Society of New York Hospitals, 211 NYT 125, 105 NE 92 (1914); Wells vs Van Nort, 100 Ohio St. 101, 125 NE 910 (1919). The principle which supports the doctrine of informed consent is that only the patient has the right to weigh the risks attending the particular treatment and decide for himself what course of action is best suited for him."

1981: Matter of Storar 52 NY 2d 363. New York.

https://casetext.com/case/matter-of-storar-2

"To the extent that existing statutory and decisional law manifests the State's interest on the subject, they consistently support the right of the competent adult to make his own decision by imposing civil liability on those who perform medical treatment without consent, although the treatment may be beneficial or even necessary to preserve the patient's life." [3 cases cited].

1982: Zant vs Prevatte. 286 SE 2d. 715, 717. Georgia.

https://law.justia.com/cases/georgia/supreme-court/1982/38375-1.html

A prison inmate had the right to starve himself by refusing forced feedings, due to his right to privacy.

"A prisoner does not relinquish his constitutional right to privacy because of his status as a prisoner. The State has no right to monitor this man's physical condition against his will; neither does it have the right to feed him to prevent his death from starvation if that is his wish. . . . it has no right to destroy a person's will by frustrating his attempt to die if necessary to make a point."

1983: Taft vs Taft. 446 NE 2d. 395. Massachusetts.

https://law.justia.com/cases/massachusetts/supreme-court/1983/388-mass-331-2.html

A woman's pregnancy required sutures to preserve the pregnancy, but this was refused by the woman on account of religious beliefs. The court upheld the woman's refusal.

"The wife's constitutional rights are established on the record. Any interest the State may have in requiring a competent, adult woman to submit to the operation is not established."

1984: Bartling vs Superior Court. 209. California Reporter 220, 225.

https://law.justia.com/cases/california/court-of-appeal/3d/163/186.html

"The right of a competent adult patient to refuse medical treatment has its origins in the constitutional right of privacy. This right is specifically guaranteed by the California Constitution (Article 1 § 1) and has been found to exist in the 'penumbra' of rights guaranteed by the Fifth and Ninth Amendments to the United States Constitution. (Griswold vs Connecticut 1965). In short the law recognizes the individual interest in preserving 'the inviolability of the person.' The constitutional right of privacy guarantees to the individual the freedom to choose to reject, or refuse to consent to, intrusions of his bodily integrity."

" . . . if the right of the patient to self-determination as to his own medical treatment is to have any meaning at all, it must be paramount to the interests of the patient's hospital and doctors. [To do otherwise] removes his freedom of choice and invades his right to self-determination." (Satz vs Perlmutter).

1985: In re Brown. 478 So. 2d 1033, 1040. Mississippi.

https://law.justia.com/cases/mississippi/supreme-court/1985/478-so-2d-1033-0.html

"The informed consent rule rests upon the bedrock of this state's respect for the individual's right to be free of unwanted bodily intrusions, no matter how well intentioned. Informed consent further suggests a corollary: the patient must be informed of the nature, means and likely consequences of the proposed treatment so that he may 'knowingly' determine what he should do, one of his options being rejection. That we would hesitate hardly a moment before holding liable a physician or hospital which proceeded without the patient's informed consent says much regarding the patient's broad right to refuse treatment."

1985: St. Mary's Hospital vs Ramsey. 465 So. 2d. 666, 668. Florida Appellate Court.

https://casetext.com/case/st-marys-hosp-v-ramsey

A Jehovah's Witness kidney patient refused a blood transfusion.

The Court ruled:

"This competent, sick adult has the right to refuse a transfusion regardless of whether his refusal to do so arises from fear of adverse reaction, religious belief, recalcitrance or cost."

1985: Matter of Conroy. 486 A 2d. 1209, 1225. New Jersey.

https://law.justia.com/cases/new-jersey/supreme-court/1985/98-n-j-321-0.html

"On balance, the right to self-determination ordinarily outweighs any countervailing state interests, and competent persons generally are permitted to refuse medical treatment, even at the risk of death."

" . . . We hold that life-sustaining treatment may be withheld or withdrawn from an incompetent patient when it is clear that the particular patient would have refused the treatment under the circumstances involved. The standard we are enunciating is a subjective one, consistent with the notion that the right that we are seeking to effectuate is a very personal right to control one's own life. The question is not what a reasonable or average person would have chosen to do under the circumstances but what the particular patient would have done if able to choose for himself."

1986: Bouvia vs Superior Court. 225 California Reporter 297 (Cal. App).

https://law.justia.com/cases/california/court-of-appeal/3d/179/1127.html

A quadriplegic expressed the wish to be allowed to die.

"The right to refuse medical treatment is basic and fundamental. It is recognized as a part of the right of privacy protected by both the state and federal constitutions. . . . . Its exercise requires no one's approval. It is not merely one vote subject to being overridden by medical opinion." [Citing Griswold vs Connecticut and Bartling vs Superior Court] are but a few examples of the decisions that have upheld a patient's right to refuse medical treatment even at risk to his health or his very life."

This decision was approved by the Conservatorship of Wendland, 28 P.3d 151, 159. California in 2001.

"But if additional persuasion be needed, there is ample. As indicated by the discussion in Bartling and Barber, substantial and respectable authority throughout the country recognize the right which petitioner seeks to exercise. Indeed, it is neither radical nor startlingly new. It is a basic and constitutionally predicated right. More than 70 years ago, Judge Benjamin Cardozo observed: 'Every human being of adult years and sound mind has a right to determine what shall be done with his own body...' (Schloendorff vs Society of New York Hospital)."

1987: In re Milton. 505 NE 2d. 255. Ohio.

https://casetext.com/case/in-re-milton-10

The State of Ohio attempted to compel an inmate of a mental hospital, who was diagnosed with psychotic delusion, to undergo treatment for a cancerous tumor.

"Appellant has expressed a long-standing belief in spiritual healing, and great weight must be given to her statement of her personal beliefs. We cannot evaluate the "correctness" or propriety of appellant's belief. Absent the most exigent circumstances, court should never be a party to branding a citizen's religious views as baseless on the grounds that they are non-traditional, unorthodox or at war with what the state or others perceive as reality."

" . . . we hold that the state may not compel a legally competent adult to submit to a medical treatment which would violate that individual's religious beliefs even though the treatment is arguably life-extending."

1987: Matter of Farrell. 529 A 2d. 404, 413. New Jersey.

https://law.justia.com/cases/new-jersey/supreme-court/1987/108-n-j-335-0.html

"Generally, a competent informed patient's 'interest in freedom from nonconsensual invasion of her bodily integrity would outweigh any state interest.' Conroy 98 New Jersey at 355, 486. A 2d, 1209, at 1226 New Jersey 1985."

"A competent patient's right to exercise his or her choice to refuse life-sustaining treatment does not vary depending on whether the patient is in a medical institution or at home."

1987: Public Health Trust of Dade County vs Wons. 500 So 2d 679 Florida Appellate Court.

https://law.justia.com/cases/florida/supreme-court/1989/69970-0.html

The Court ruled that the State's interest in having children reared by two parents was not a sufficient reason to order a Jehovah's Witness patient to submit to a blood transfusion.

"By forcing Mrs. Wons to submit to a blood transfusion forbidden by her religious beliefs, the state compelled rather than prohibited affirmative conduct, and there was no immediate public danger posed by her refusal to consent to the transfusion. Therefore, cases concerning the prohibition of affirmative religiously based conduct are inapposite to this case." (See in re Estate of Brooks).

1987: Sagala vs Tavares. 367 Pennsylvania Superior Court 573, 578, 533 A 2d 165, 167

https://cite.case.law/pa-super/367/573/#p578

"In order for a consent to be considered informed it must be shown that the patient was advised of 'those risks which a reasonable man would have considered material to his decision whether or not to undergo treatment.' " (Cooper vs Roberts 220 PA Super 260, 286A 2d. 647.)
And that this is the standard of care. (Festa vs Greenberg, 354 PA Superior Court 346, 511 A 2d 1371, 1373. 1986)

"As a practical matter, an operation performed without informed consent is a technical battery, which makes the physician liable for any injuries resulting from that invasion."

1988: Cruzan vs Harmon. 760 SW 2nd, 408, 417. Missouri.

https://law.justia.com/cases/missouri/supreme-court/1988/70813-0.html

"The doctrine of informed consent arose in recognition of the value society places on a person's autonomy and as the primary vehicle by which a person can protect the integrity of his body. If one can consent to treatment, one can also refuse it. Thus, as a necessary corollary to informed consent, the right to refuse treatment arose."

"A decision as to medical treatment must be informed."

"There are three basic prerequisites for informed consent: the patient must have the capacity to reason and make judgments, the decision must be made voluntarily and without coercion, and the patient must have a clear understanding of the risks and benefits of the proposed treatment alternatives or nontreatment, along with a full understanding of the nature of the disease and the prognosis."

1989: In re EG, 549 NE 2d 322, 328 Illinois.

https://law.justia.com/cases/illinois/supreme-court/1989/66089-7.html

A 17-year old leukemia patient and Jehovah's Witness refused blood transfusion, upheld by the court.

"We find that a mature minor may exercise a common law right to consent to or refuse medical care...."

"Because we find that a mature minor may exercise a common law right to consent to or refuse medical care, we decline to address the constitutional issue."

1990: In re Guardianship of Browning. 568 So 2nd 4, 10 Florida.

https://law.justia.com/cases/florida/supreme-court/1990/74174-0.html

"An integral component of self-determination is the right to make choices pertaining to one's health, including the right to refuse unwanted medical treatment."

"Recognizing that one has the inherent right to make choices about medical treatment, we necessarily conclude that this right encompasses all medical choices. A competent individual has the constitutional right to refuse medical treatment regardless of his or her medical condition. . . . The issue involves a patient's right of self-determination and does not involve what is thought to be in the patient's best interests."

1990: In re AC., 573 A 2d. 1235, 1252. Washington DC 1990, en banc.

https://law.justia.com/cases/district-of-columbia/court-of-appeals/1990/87-609-4.html

" . . . the right of bodily integrity is not extinguished simply because someone is ill, or even at death's door. To protect that right against intrusion by others, family members, doctors, hospitals, or anyone else, however, well-intentioned, we hold that a court must determine the patient's wishes by any means available, and must abide by those wishes unless there are truly extraordinary or compelling reasons to override them."

"We emphasize, nevertheless, that it would be an extraordinary case indeed in which a court might ever be justified in overriding the patient's wishes and authorizing a major surgical procedure such as a caesarian section. Throughout this opinion we have stressed that the patient's wishes, once they are ascertained must be followed in 'virtually all cases,' ante at 1249, unless there are 'truly extraordinary or compelling reasons to override them,' ante at 1247. Indeed, some may doubt that there could ever be a situation extraordinary or compelling enough to justify a massive intrusion into a person's body, such as a caesarean section, against that person's will."

1990: Cruzan vs Director, Missouri Dept of Health. 497 US 261, 270.

https://www.law.cornell.edu/supremecourt/text/497/261

This US Supreme Court case has been cited as the definitive case that prohibits government / police power enforcement of any medical treatment.

"The logical corollary of the doctrine of informed consent is that the patient generally possesses the right not to consent, that is, to refuse treatment."

"Most state courts have based a right to refuse treatment on the common law right to informed consent, see e.g. In re Storar or on both that right and a constitutional privacy right see e.g. Superintendent of Belchertown State School vs Saikewicz."

1991: Norwood Hospital vs Muñoz: 564 NE 2d 1017, Massachusetts.

http://masscases.com/cases/sjc/409/409mass116.html

A Jehovah's Witness, who was the mother of a minor child, had a right to refuse blood transfusion, upheld by the Court.

"A competent adult has a common law and constitutional right to refuse a life-saving blood transfusion, based on the individual's rights to bodily integrity and privacy. . . . There is no doubt, therefore, that Ms. Muñoz has a right to refuse the blood transfusion."

1992: Matter of Guardianship of LW. 481 NW 2d 60, 65. Wisconsin.

https://law.justia.com/cases/wisconsin/supreme-court/1992/89-1197-9.html

"The logical corollary of the doctrine of informed consent is the right not to consent – the right to refuse treatment."
"We conclude that an individual's right to refuse unwanted medical treatment emanates from the common law right of self-determination and informed consent, the personal liberties protected by the Fourteenth Amendment and from the guarantee of liberty in Article 1 Section 1 of the Wisconsin Constitution."

1993: Thor vs Superior Court. 855 P. 2d. 375. California.

https://law.justia.com/cases/california/supreme-court/4th/5/725.html

"More than a century ago, the United States Supreme Court declared, "No right is held more sacred, or is more carefully guarded, by the common law, than the right of every individual to possession and control of his own person, free from all restraint or interference of others, unless by clear and unquestionable authority of law. . . . 'The right to one's person may be said to be a right of complete immunity: to be let alone.' [Citation.]" (Union Pacific Railway Co. vs Botsford 1891)."

"Until recently, the question of a patient's right to refuse life-sustaining treatment has implicated potentially conflicting medical, legal and ethical considerations. The developing interdisciplinary consensus, however, now uniformly recognizes the patient's right of control over bodily integrity as the subsuming essential in determining the relative balance of interests. . . . This preeminent deference derives principally from 'the long-standing importance in our Anglo-American legal tradition of personal autonomy and the right of self-determination.' [5 cases cited]. As John Stuart Mill succinctly stated, 'Over himself, over his own body and mind, the individual is sovereign.' Mill, On Liberty (1859 p. 13).

"Because health care decisions intrinsically concern one's subjective sense of well-being, this right of personal autonomy does not turn on the wisdom, i.e., medical rationality, of the individual's choice."

"We therefore hold that Andrews's right of self-determination and bodily integrity prevails over any countervailing duty to preserve life."

1996: In re Fiori. 673. A. 2d. 905, 910. Pennsylvania.

https://cite.case.law/pa/543/592/

"From this right to be free from bodily invasion developed the doctrine of informed consent. (See Schloendorff.) The doctrine of informed consent declares that absent an emergency situation, medical treatment may not be imposed without the patient's informed consent. A logical corollary to this doctrine is the patient's right, in general, 'to refuse treatment and to withdraw consent to treatment once begun.' Courts have unanimously concluded that this right to self-determination does not cease upon the incapacitation of the individual." [3 cases cited]

2001: In re Duran. 769 A 2d 497. Pennsylvania Superior Court.

https://law.justia.com/cases/pennsylvania/superior-court/2001/a02026-01.html

Liver transplant patient gave explicit instructions not to receive transfused blood during operation.

"Appellant next argues that the trial court violated Maria's common law and constitutional rights when it appointed an emergency guardian to consent to a blood transfusion on behalf of Maria in spite of her religious beliefs and prior directives. We agree."

"[The patient's] unequivocal refusal of blood transfusion therapy is protected by Pennsylvania common law and that the trial court erred when it appointed an emergency guardian to abridge this right."

"The right to refuse medical treatment is deeply rooted in our common law. This right to bodily integrity was recognized by the United States Supreme Court over a century ago when it proclaimed 'no right is held more sacred, or is more carefully guarded by the common law, than the right of every individual to the possession and control of his own person . . . .' " (Union Pacific Railway Co vs Botsford.)

"The right to control the integrity of one's body spawned the doctrine of informed consent." (See Fiori; Schloendorff)

2001: Conservatorship of Wendland. 28 P 3d. 151, 158. California.

https://law.justia.com/cases/california/supreme-court/4th/26/519.html

"One relatively certain principle is that a competent adult has the right to refuse medical treatment, even treatment necessary to sustain life. The Legislature has cited this principle to justify legislation governing medical care decisions (§ 4650), and courts have invoked it as a starting point for [26 Cal. 4th 531] analysis, even in cases examining the rights of incompetent persons and the duties of surrogate decision makers." [2 cases cited].

2008: Salandy vs Bryk. 864 New York 2d 46 New York AD.

https://casetext.com/case/salandy-v-bryk

A Jehovah's Witness patient refused a blood transfusion, however the physician ignored the patient and performed the transfusion. The Court held that the patient could sue the physician for medical malpractice and infliction of emotional distress.

2010: Stouffer vs. Reid. 993 A 2nd 104, 109. Maryland.

https://casetext.com/case/stouffer-v-reid-1

"We explained that the 'fountainhead of the doctrine [of informed consent] is the patient's right to exercise control over his own body . . . by deciding for himself [or herself] whether or not to submit to the particular therapy.' (Mack, 618 A 2d at 755. Maryland; Sard vs Hardy. 379 A 2d 1014, 1019. Maryland.) Further, we point out that 'a corollary to the doctrine is the patient's right, in general, to refuse treatment and to withdraw consent to treatment once begun.'" Id.

Even persons who are confined in the State's custody have a constitutional right to refuse "treatment," at least in some situations. (Davis vs Hubbard). See for example, **Mackey vs Procunier**, 477 F 2d 877 (9th Circuit 1973); **Knecht vs Gillman**, 488 F. 2d 1136 (8th Cir. 1973); **Scott vs Plante**, 532 F 2d 939 (3rd Cir. 1976); **Bell vs Wayne County General Hospital**, 384 F. Supp. 1085, 1100 ED Mich. 1974); **Rennie vs Klein**, 462 F Supp. 1131 (D NJ 1978); **Rogers vs Okin**, 478 F Supp. 1342 (D. Mass 1979)

Two very pertinent and famous cases are notably missing from this list of cases.

Roe vs Wade addressed bodily autonomy and self-determination of a pregnant woman. What has remained controversial is to what extent the other human being contained within her body is or is not also endowed with, or may have claim to, the rights of people, such as life. I leave that complex and long-debated matter (back to at least the time of Aristotle) for other discussions in different venues.

The other pertinent and controversial case in this area of bodily autonomy is the much misunderstood and misquoted Jacobson vs Massachusetts case of 1905.

https://supreme.justia.com/cases/federal/us/197/11/

Mr. Jacobson had nearly died as a child after receiving a smallpox vaccine in his native Europe. Later, having immigrated to the US, the State of Massachusetts sought to compel citizens to receive a smallpox vaccine. Jacobson prosecuted the State. The US Supreme Court favored the belief that smallpox vaccination was safe and effective, and therefore there was a compelling state interest in mandating the injection on citizens.

Justice John Marshall Harlan, writing for the majority:

"Until otherwise informed by the highest court of Massachusetts we are not inclined to hold that the statute establishes the absolute rule that an adult must be vaccinated if it be apparent or can be shown with reasonable certainty that he is not at the time a fit subject of vaccination or that vaccination, by reason of his then condition, would seriously impair his health or probably cause his death. No such case is here presented."

However, it had already been empirically observed for over twenty years, since the Leicester England tragedies, that those vaccinated with smallpox were more likely to die of smallpox than the unvaccinated, and that stricter smallpox vaccination laws in the 1860's were followed by an acceleration of smallpox outbreaks, until a smallpox pandemic swept through Europe in 1870-1872. Journalists, professors, doctors and parents warned of outbreaks following – not preceding – vaccination campaigns. [356]

What is little known about the 1905 Jacobson case is that Jacobson was given a choice to pay a five-dollar fine or to submit to the vaccination, and Jacobson ultimately chose to pay the fine. This would be about $ 161.20 in today's currency.

"And the Court ordered that he stand committed until the fine was paid."

The US Supreme Court did not mandate the government or police to force Mr. Jacobson to have the vaccine against his will. But they did fine him for this decision.

Was Jacobson unreasonable in his refusal to be vaccinated?

Twenty years earlier in Leicester England during a demonstration of 80,000 to 100,000 people from all over England, Mr. Councillor Butcher of Leicester said of the mass of people who had gathered,

"They lived for something else in this world than to be experimented upon for the stamping out of a particular disease. A large and increasing portion of the public were of the opinion that the best way to get rid of smallpox and similar diseases was to use plenty of water, eat good food, live in light and airy houses, and see that the Corporation kept the streets clean and the drains in order. If such details were attended to, there was no need to fear smallpox, or any of its kindred; and if they were neglected, neither vaccination nor any other prescription by Act of Parliament could save them." [357]

Dedication

I would like to repeat that this book is dedicated to
Ernesto Ramirez, Jr.
who lost his life,
at 16 years old, just 5 days after his first Pfizer vaccine,
an event verified on autopsy by four independent physicians,
although Ernesto played sports and had no health problems before
the vaccine.   Here Ernest's Dad lays to rest his son.

Ernest Ramirez
@rgvrunner01

My good byes to my Baby Boy 💔💔💔

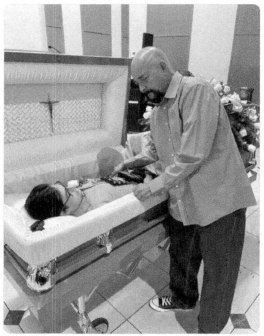

7:44 PM · Sep 13, 2021 · Twitter for iPhone

This book is also dedicated to all those who lost loved ones
following vaccines, or who tried to talk a loved one out of a vaccine,
or who risked their source of income or their education, standing
strong against peer pressure, bullying, superstition and
"mandates."

Endnotes

Chapter 1: Danger signals from human and animal studies

[1] FDA Briefing Document: Pfizer-BioNTech COVID-19 Vaccine. Vaccines and related biological products advisory committee meeting. Dec 10 2020. Sponsor: Pfizer and BioNTech. https://www.fda.gov/media/144245/download

[2] FDA. Emergency use authorization of medical products and related authorities. Jan 2017. https://www.fda.gov/regulatory-information/search-fda-guidance-documents/emergency-use-authorization-medical-products-and-related-authorities

[3] C Huber. The Defeat of COVID. Apr 10 2021. https://www.amazon.com/Defeat-COVID-medical-studies-doesnt/dp/0578248212/ref=sr_1_1

[4] J Ioannidis. Reconciling estimates of global spread and infection fatality rates of COVID-19: An overview of systematic evaluations. Mar 26 2021. https://onlinelibrary.wiley.com/doi/10.1111/eci.13554

[5] A Ault. Can a COVID-19 vaccine stop the spread? Good question. Nov 20 2020. Medscape. https://www.medscape.com/viewarticle/941388

[6] I Kershner. Israel, once the model for beating Covid, faces new surge of infections. Oct 3 2021 NY Times. https://www.nytimes.com/2021/08/18/world/middleeast/israel-virus-infections-booster.html

[7] FDA Briefing Document: Pfizer-BioNTech COVID-19 Vaccine. Vaccines and related biological products advisory committee meeting. Dec 10 2020. Sponsor: Pfizer and BioNTech. P 42. https://www.fda.gov/media/144245/download

[8] H Vennema, R de Groot, et al. Early death after feline infectious peritonitis virus challenge due to recombinant vaccinia virus immunization. Mar 1990. J Virol. 64 (3). 1407-1409. https://www.ncbi.nlm.nih.gov/pmc/articles/PMC249267/

[9] H Weingarti, M Czub, et al. Immunization with modified vaccinia virus Ankara-based recombinant vaccine against severe acute respiratory syndrome is associated with enhanced hepatitis in ferrets. Nov 2004 J Virol. 78 (22). https://www.ncbi.nlm.nih.gov/pmc/articles/PMC525089/

[10] S Gold, J Todaro, et al. America's Frontline Doctors' White Paper on experimental vaccines for COVID-19. https://img1.wsimg.com/blobby/go/99d35b02-a5cb-41e6-ad80-a070f8a5ee17/SMDwhitepaper.pdf

[11] C Tseng, E Sbrana, et al. Immunization with SARS coronavirus vaccines leads to pulmonary immunopathology on challenge with the SARS virus. Apr 20 2012. PLoS One. 7 (4). https://www.ncbi.nlm.nih.gov/pmc/articles/PMC3335060/

[12] K Wylon, S Dolle, et al. Polyethylene glycol as a cause of anaphylaxis. Dec 13 2016. Allergy Asthma & Clin Immun. 12 (67). https://aacijournal.biomedcentral.com/articles/10.1186/s13223-016-0172-7

[13] Kyodo News. Japan sees high rate of anaphylaxis after taking Pfizer vaccine. Mar 10 2021. https://english.kyodonews.net/news/2021/03/a31eccc9b9e3-japan-sees-high-rate-of-anaphylaxis-after-taking-pfizer-vaccine.html

[14] US Centers for Disease Control and Prevention (CDC). Vaccines and immunizations. Last updated Feb 11 2022. https://www.cdc.gov/vaccines/covid-19/clinical-considerations/managing-anaphylaxis.html

[15] S Zhang, Y Xu, et al. Cationic compounds used in lipoplexes and polyplexes for gene delivery. Nov 24 2004. J Cont Release. 100 (2). https://www.sciencedirect.com/science/article/abs/pii/S0168365904004006?via%3Dihub

[16] S Dokka, D Toledo, et al. Oxygen radical-mediated pulmonary toxicity induced by some cationic liposomes. May 2000. Pharm Res. https://pubmed.ncbi.nlm.nih.gov/10888302/

[17] S Cui, Y Wang, et al. Correlation of the cytotoxic effects of cationic lipids with their headgroups. Mar 22 2018. Toxicol Res. https://pubmed.ncbi.nlm.nih.gov/30090597/

[18] H Lv, S Zhang, et al. Toxicity of cationic lipids and cationic polymers in gene delivery. Aug 10 2006. J Control Release. https://pubmed.ncbi.nlm.nih.gov/16831482/

[19] C Lonez, M Lensink, et al. Interaction between cationic lipids and endotoxin receptors. Feb 1 2009. Biophysical J. https://www.cell.com/biophysj/fulltext/S0006-3495(08)03808-3#relatedArticles

[20] M Zhang, J Sun, et al. Modified mRNA-LNP vaccines confer protection against experimental DENV-2 infection in mice. Sept 11 2020. Mol Ther Meth & Clin Dev. 18 (11).
https://www.sciencedirect.com/science/article/pii/S2329050120301625

[21] F Arkin. Dengue vaccine fiasco leads to criminal charges for researcher in the Philippines. Apr 24 2019. Science.
https://www.science.org/content/article/dengue-vaccine-fiasco-leads-criminal-charges-researcher-philippines

[22] L Zhang, A Richards, et al. SARS-CoV-2 RNA reverse-transcribed and integrated into the human genome. Dec 13 2020. bioRxiv.
https://pubmed.ncbi.nlm.nih.gov/33330870/

[23] T Buzhdygan, B DeOre, et al. The SARS-CoV-2 spike protein alters barrier function in 2D static and microfluidic models of the human blood-brain barrier. Dec 2020. Nuerobiol Dis. 146.
https://www.ncbi.nlm.nih.gov/pmc/articles/PMC7547916/

[24] Medical Xpress. SARS-CoV-2 spike protein alone may cause lung damage. Interview with Pavle Solopov, PhD, DVM. Apr 27 2021.
https://medicalxpress.com/news/2021-04-sars-cov-spike-protein-lung.html

[25] Y Lei, J Zhang, et al. SARS-CoV-2 spike protein impairs endothelial function via downregulation of ACE2. Mar 31 2021. Circulation Research. 128 (9).
https://www.ahajournals.org/doi/10.1161/CIRCRESAHA.121.318902

[26] W Lee, A Wheatley, et al. Antibody-dependent enhancement and SARS-CoV-2 vaccines and therapies. Sep 9 2020. Nature Microbiology.
https://www.nature.com/articles/s41564-020-00789-5

[27] T Hohdatsu, M Nakamuyra, et al. A study on the mechanism of antibody-dependent enhancement of feline infectious peritonitis virus infection in feline macrophages by monoclonal antibodies. 1991. Arch Virol. 120 (3-4).
https://pubmed.ncbi.nlm.nih.gov/1659798/

[28] R Weiss, F Scott. Antibody-mediated enhancement of disease in feline infectious peritonitis: comparisons with dengue hemorrhagic fever. 1981. Comp Immunol Microbiol Infect Dis. 4 (2).
https://pubmed.ncbi.nlm.nih.gov/6754243/

[29] C Tseng, e Sbrana, et al. Immunization with SARS coronavirus vaccines leads to pulmonary immunopathology on challenge with the SARS virus. Apr 20 2012. PLoS One. 7 (4). https://www.ncbi.nlm.nih.gov/pmc/articles/PMC3335060/

[30] S Alturki, S Alturki, et al. The 2020 pandemic: Current SARS-CoV-2 vaccine development. 2020. Front Immunol. https://www.ncbi.nlm.nih.gov/pmc/articles/PMC7466534/

[31] M Cloutier, M Nandi, et al. ADE and hyperinflammation in SARS-CoV-2 infection – comparison with dengue hemorrhagic fever and feline infectious peritonitis. Dec 2020. Cytokine. https://www.ncbi.nlm.nih.gov/pmc/articles/PMC7439999/

[32] The Exposé. MHRA data shows a 3016% increase in the number of women who've lost their unborn child as a result of having the COVID vaccine. June 16 2021. The Exposé. https://dailyexpose.uk/2021/06/16/3016-increase-loss-baby-due-covid-jab/

[33] Gov.UK. Coronavirus vaccine – weekly summary of yellow card reporting. P 82. https://assets.publishing.service.gov.uk/government/uploads/system/uploads/attachment_data/file/1072043/COVID-19_mRNA_Pfizer-_BioNTech_vaccine_analysis_print.pdf

[34] T Shimabukuro, S Kim et al. Preliminary findings of mRNA COVID-19 vaccine safety in pregnant women. Apr 21 2021. NEJM. https://www.nejm.org/doi/full/10.1056/NEJMoa2104983

[35] University of Miami, Miller School of Medicine. University of Miami researchers studying effects of COVID-19 vaccine and male fertility. Dec 18 2020. Newswise. https://www.newswise.com/coronavirus/university-of-miami-researchers-studying-effects-of-covid-19-vaccine-and-male-fertility

[36] CDC. Clinical considerations: Myocarditis and pericarditis after receipt of mRNA COVID-19 vaccines among adolescents and young adults. https://www.cdc.gov/vaccines/covid-19/clinical-considerations/myocarditis.html

[37] E Avolio, M Gamez, et al. The SARS-CoV-2 spike protein disrupts the cooperative function of human cardiac pericytes – endothelial cells through CD 147 receptor-mediated signalling: a potential non-infective mechanism of COVID-19 microvascular disease. Dec 21 2020. bioRxiv. https://www.biorxiv.org/content/10.1101/2020.12.21.423721v1

[38] C Huber. Heart damage from the COVID vaccines: Is it avoidable? July 14 2021. PDMJ. https://pdmj.org/papers/myocarditis_paper

[39] C Huber. Heart fatigue from vaccines, as shown by fluid dynamics. Jan 16 2022. The Defeat Of COVID. https://colleenhuber.substack.com/p/heart-fatigue-from-vaccines-as-shown

[40] R Hodkinson MD, interviewed on The High Wire by Del Bigtree, Episode 220. https://thehighwire.com/watch/

[41] Pfizer. A Phase 1/2/3, placebo-controlled, randomized, observer-blind, dose-finding study to evaluate the safety, tolerability, immunogenicity, and efficacy of SARS-CoV-2 RNA vaccine candidates against COVID-19 in healthy individuals. 2020. Pp 67-68. https://cdn.pfizer.com/pfizercom/2020-11/C4591001_Clinical_Protocol_Nov2020.pdf

[42] H Noorchasm. A letter of warning to FDA and Pfizer: On the immunological danger of COVID-19 vaccination in the naturally infected. Jan 26 2021, reprinted Nov 29 2021. https://citizenwells.substack.com/p/a-letter-of-warning-to-fda-and-pfizer?s=r

[43] M Sones. Vaccination in Israel: Challenging mortality figures? Interview with Dr. Hervé Seligmann. Feb 18 2021. Israel National News. https://www.israelnationalnews.com/news/297051

[44] US Code of Federal Regulations. 45 CFR § 46.116. General requirements for informed consent. https://www.law.cornell.edu/cfr/text/45/46.116

[45] Pfizer. Fact sheet for healthcare providers administering vaccine: Emergency use authorization (EUA) of the Pfizer-BioNTech COVID-19 vaccine to prevent coronavirus disease 2019 (COVID-19). https://labeling.pfizer.com/ShowLabeling.aspx

[46] Daily Med. Moderna COVID-19 vaccine- cx024414 injection, suspension. https://dailymed.nlm.nih.gov/dailymed/drugInfo.cfm

[47] T Beer. Large numbers of health care and frontline workers are refusing COVID-19 vaccine. Jan 2 2021. https://www.forbes.com/sites/tommybeer/2021/01/02/large-numbers-of-health-care-and-frontline-workers-are-refusing-covid-19-vaccine/

[48] A Siri. Federal law prohibits employers and others from requiring vaccination with a COVID-19 vaccine distributed under an EUA. Feb 23 2021. STAT.

https://www.statnews.com/2021/02/23/federal-law-prohibits-employers-and-others-from-requiring-vaccination-with-a-covid-19-vaccine-distributed-under-an-eua/

[49] NVIC. National Vaccine Information Center. https://www.nvic.org/

[50] Children's Health Defense. https://childrenshealthdefense.org/

[51] Informed Consent Action Network (ICAN). https://www.icandecide.org/

[52] A Powe. Exclusive with Dr Peter McCullough. 'Don't take any more' genetic vaccines, dangerous foreign spike proteins [which] 'lead to chronic disease.' Jan 24 2022. https://www.thegatewaypundit.com/2022/01/exclusive-dr-peter-mccullough-urges-stand-genetic-vaccines-cause-body-produce-spike-proteins-brain-lung-heart-bone-marrow-reproductive-organs/

[53] M Fauzia. Fact check: FDA did not associate Pfizer's first vaccine dose with COVID-19 infections. Apr 27 2021. USA Today. https://www.usatoday.com/story/news/factcheck/2021/04/27/fact-check-false-claim-fda-and-pfizers-first-vaccine-dose/7188089002/

[54] Life Site News. Yale public health professor suggests 60% of new COVID-19 patients have received vaccine. Apr 21 2021. LifeSite News. https://www.lifesitenews.com/news/yale-public-health-professor-suggests-60-of-new-covid-19-patients-have-received-vaccine/

[55] CDC. When you've been fully vaccinated. Updated Oct 15 2021. https://www.cdc.gov/coronavirus/2019-ncov/vaccines/fully-vaccinated_archived.html

Chapter 2: Court testimony on the COVID vaccines

[56] P McCullough. Safety First lecture; video segment Apr 16 2022. Twitter. https://twitter.com/p_mcculloughmd/status/1515430172052398092?s=21&t=EOU1jFUP6JZn9d_cHT2WRQ

[57] US Centers for Disease Control and Prevention. National Vital Statistics System. State and national provisional counts. Monthly and 12-month ending number of live births, deaths and infant deaths: United States. https://www.cdc.gov/nchs/nvss/vsrr/provisional-tables.htm

[58] Ibid.

[59] BioNTech. US Securities and Exchange Commission. Form 20-F Annual Report. Mar 30 2022. P 6. https://investors.biontech.de/static-files/50d0cafc-b2c1-4392-a495-d252f84be105

[60] K Beattie. Worldwide Bayesian causal impact analysis of vaccine administration on deaths and cases associated with COVID-19: A big data analysis of 145 countries. Preprint. Nov 15 2021. https://drive.google.com/file/d/1DLlRa9rUqvW9pG1vNEsWMEydWwsmSMbe/view

[61] Ibid. 41.

[62] Ibid. 39.

[63] C Hansen, A Schelde, et al. Vaccine effectiveness against SARS-CoV-2 infection with the Omicron or Delta variants following a two-dose or booster BNT162b2 or mRNA-1273 vaccination series: A Danish cohort study. https://www.medrxiv.org/content/10.1101/2021.12.20.21267966v3.full.pdf

[64] Status of the SARS-CoV-2 variant Omicron in Denmark. COVID-19 Omicron variant report. Dec 31 2021. Statens Serum Institut. https://files.ssi.dk/covid19/omikron/statusrapport/rapport-omikronvarianten-31122021-ct18

[65] Office for National Statistics. Coronavirus (COVID-19) infection survey, UK: Characteristics related to having an Omicron compatible result in those who test positive for COVID-19. Dec 21 2021. https://www.ons.gov.uk/peoplepopulationandcommunity/healthandsocialcare/conditionsanddiseases/adhocs/14107coronaviruscovid19infectionsurveyukcharacteristicsrelatedtohavinganomicroncompatibleresultinthosewhotestpositiveforcovid19

[66] UK Health Security Agency. COVID-19 vaccine surveillance report. Week 9. Mar 3 2022. https://assets.publishing.service.gov.uk/government/uploads/system/uploads/attachment_data/file/1058464/Vaccine-surveillance-report-week-9.pdf

[67] UK Office for National Statistics. Death by vaccination status, England. https://www.ons.gov.uk/peoplepopulationandcommunity/birthsdeathsandmarriages/deaths/datasets/deathsbyvaccinationstatusengland

Gov.UK no longer shows Table 9, as of May 17 2022. I re-write the tables on p 33 here:
Table 9, ONS Report: Whole period causes of deaths and person-years by vaccination status and five year age group, England, deaths occurring between 1 January 2021 and October 2021.

Vaccination status	Age group	Person-years	Deaths involving COVID-19	Non-COVID-19 deaths	All deaths
Received only the first dose, at least 21 days ago	10-14	6,618	0	3	3
	15-19	174,657	0	32	32
Received the second dose, at least 21 days ago	10-14	1,678	0	4	4
	15-19	127,342	1	41	42
Unvaccinated	10-14	2,034,711	2	94	96
	15-19	1,547,072	18	142	160

[68] Lifesite News. British children are up to 52 times more likely to die following a COVID shot. Feb 2 2022. https://www.lifesitenews.com/news/children-in-britain-up-to-52-times-more-likely-to-die-following-a-covid-shot-report-finds/

[69] J Horgan-Jones. The Irish Times. Jan 22 2022. Total of 100,000 Covid vaccines expire amid slowing demand, Ministers told. https://www.irishtimes.com/news/ireland/irish-news/total-of-100-000-covid-vaccines-expire-amid-slowing-demand-ministers-told-1.4782708

[70] Public Health Scotland. Public Health Scotland COVID-19 & Winter Statistical Report. Jan 17 2022. https://publichealthscotland.scot/media/11802/22-01-19-covid19-winter_publication_report_revised.pdf

[71] Public Health Scotland. Births and babies: Infant deaths. Apr 17 2022. https://scotland.shinyapps.io/phs-covid-wider-impact/

[72] Johns Hopkins University. Our World in Data. https://ourworldindata.org/coronavirus#explore-the-global-situation

[73] Robert Koch Institut. COVID-19 in Germany. https://www.rki.de/EN/Home/homepage_node.html

[74] Wochentlicher Lagebericht des RKI zur Coronavirus-Krankheit-2019 (COVID-19) [article in German] Dec 30 2021. Robert Koch Institut. https://www.rki.de/DE/Content/InfAZ/N/Neuartiges_Coronavirus/Situationsberichte/Wochenbericht/Wochenbericht_2021-12-30.pdf?__blob=publicationFile

[75] El gato malo. German Omicron Data. Dec 31 2021.
https://boriquagato.substack.com/p/german-omicron-data

[76] R Steyer, G Kappler. The higher the vaccination rate, the higher the excess mortality. Nov 16 2021. https://www.skirsch.com/covid/GermanAnalysis.pdf
https://www.utebergner.de/cms/wp-content/uploads/2021/11/%C3%9Cbersterblichkeit-KW-36-bis-40-in-2021-003.docx

[77] G Kampf. COVID-19 stigmatising the unvaccinated is not justified. Nov 20 2021. The Lancet. 398: 10314. P 1871.
https://www.thelancet.com/journals/lancet/article/PIIS0140-6736(21)02243-1/fulltext

[78] A Dutt. Out of 34 Omicron cases at Delhi hospital, 33 are fully vaccinated. The Indian Express. Dec 23 2021.
https://indianexpress.com/article/cities/delhi/out-of-34-omicron-cases-at-delhi-hospital-33-are-fully-vaccinated-7686188/

[79] T Lambert. 99.6% of COVID deaths in Canada were among vaccinated people between April 10-17. May 6 2022. The Counter Signal.
https://thecountersignal.com/99-per-cent-covid-deaths-in-canada-among-vaccinated/

[80] Government of Canada. Archive Today. Updated Apr 17 2022.
https://archive.ph/EdHxU

[81] Government of Canada. COVID-19 vaccination in Canada. Updated Apr 29 2022. https://health-infobase.canada.ca/covid-19/vaccination-coverage/

[82] Pfizer Worldwide Safety. 5.3.6 Cumulative analysis of post-authorization adverse event reports of PF-07302048 (BNT162B2) received through 28 Feb 2021. P 7. https://phmpt.org/wp-content/uploads/2021/11/5.3.6-postmarketing-experience.pdf

[83] Public Health and Medical Professionals for Transparency Documents vs Food and Drug Administration. Complaint for Declaratory and Injunctive Relief. Sep 16 2021. US District Court, Northern District of Texas. https://phmpt.org/wp-content/uploads/2021/10/001-Complaint-101021.pdf

[84] Public Health and Medical Professionals for Transparency Documents.
https://phmpt.org/wp-content/uploads/2021/11/5.3.6-postmarketing-experience.pdf

[85] Celia Farber. Court-ordered Pfizer documents they tried to have sealed for 55 years show 1223 deaths, 158,000 adverse events in 90 days post EUA release. Dec 5 2021. https://celiafarber.substack.com/p/court-ordered-pfizer-documents-they?utm_source=substack&utm_campaign=post_embed&utm_medium=web

[86] Canadian COVID Care Alliance. The Pfizer inoculations for COVID-19: More harm than good. https://www.canadiancovidcarealliance.org/wp-content/uploads/2021/12/The-COVID-19-Inoculations-More-Harm-Than-Good-REV-Dec-16-2021.pdf

[87] US Department of Health and Human Services. Vaccine Adverse Event Reporting System (VAERS). https://vaers.hhs.gov/
[88] Open VAERS. COVID vaccine data. https://openvaers.com/covid-data/mortality

[89] US Department of Health and Human Services. Vaccine Adverse Event Reporting System (VAERS). https://vaers.hhs.gov/

[90] Open VAERS. COVID vaccine data. https://openvaers.com/covid-data/mortality

[91] The Exposé. Study finds COVID-19 vaccination increases risk of suffering a stroke by 11,361%. May 2 2022. https://dailyexpose.uk/2022/05/02/study-covid-vaccines-increase-risk-stroke-11361percent/

[92] US Centers for Disease Control and Prevention. https://wonder.cdc.gov/vaers.html

[93] The Exposé. FACT: Covid-19 vaccines are almost 50 times deadlier than the flu vaccines per number of doses administered according to official USA data. Feb 21 2022. https://dailyexpose.uk/2022/02/21/covid-vaccines-50-times-deadlier-than-flu-vaccines/

[94] Centers for Disease Control and Prevention (CDC) Vaccine Adverse Event Reporting System (VAERS). https://wonder.cdc.gov/vaers.html

[95] Pfizer Worldwide Safety. 5.3.6 Cumulative analysis of post-authorization adverse event reports of PF-07302048 (BNT162B2) received through 28 Feb 2021. P 7. https://phmpt.org/wp-content/uploads/2021/11/5.3.6-postmarketing-experience.pdf

[96] J Greene. 'Paramount importance:' Judge orders FDA to hasten release of Pfizer vaccine docs. Jan 7 2022. https://www.reuters.com/legal/government/paramount-importance-judge-orders-fda-hasten-release-pfizer-vaccine-docs-2022-01-07/

[97] P Thacker. COVID-19: Researcher blows the whistle on data integrity issues in Pfizer's vaccine trial. BMJ 2021; 375. https://www.bmj.com/content/375/bmj.n2635

[98] Pfizer Worldwide Safety. 5.3.6 Cumulative analysis of post-authorization adverse event reports of PF-07302048 (BNT162B2) received through 28 Feb 2021. Appendix 1: List of adverse events of special interest. Pp 30-38. https://phmpt.org/wp-content/uploads/2021/11/5.3.6-postmarketing-experience.pdf

[99] Pfizer Worldwide Safety. Ibid.

[100] Senator Ron Johnson. Video Release: Sen. Ron Johnson COVID-19 A Second Opinion Panel garners over 800,000 views in 24 hours. Jan 25 2022. https://www.ronjohnson.senate.gov/2022/1/video-release-sen-ron-johnson-covid-19-a-second-opinion-panel-garners-over-800-000-views-in-24-hours

[101] US Navy Seals 1-26 vs Biden (4:21-cv-01236) District Court, ND Texas. https://www.courtlistener.com/docket/60824061/us-navy-seals-1-26-v-biden/

[102] S Kirsch, J Rose, M Crawford. Estimating the number of COVID vaccine deaths in America. Dec 24 2021. https://www.skirsch.com/covid/Deaths.pdf

[103] S Kirsch. Latest VAERS estimate: 388,000 Americans killed by the COVID vaccines. Dec 14 2021. Steve Kirsch's Newsletter. https://stevekirsch.substack.com/p/latest-vaers-estimate-388000-americans

[104] How much more evidence do you need? https://elcolectivodeuno.wordpress.com/2021/12/29/how-much-more-evidence-do-you-need-here-is-a-list-of-860-scientific-studies-and-reports-linking-covid-vaccines-to-hundreds-of-adverse-effects-and-deaths/

[105] S Kirsch. Interview: Rheumatologist Robert Jackson: 40% of my 3,000 vaccinated patients report a significant vaccine injury. May 1 2022. Steve Kirsch's Newsletter. https://stevekirsch.substack.com/p/rheumatologist-robert-jackson-40

[106] P Machado, S Lawson-Tovey, et al. Safety of vaccination against SARS-CoV-2 in people with rheumatic and musculoskeletal diseases: results from the EULAR Coronavirus Vaccine (COVAX) physician-reported registry. Dec 31 2021. Ann Rheum Dis. https://ard.bmj.com/content/81/5/695

[107] S Bhakdi, A Burkhardt. On COVID vaccines: why they cannot work, and irrefutable evidence of their causative role in deaths after vaccination. https://doctors4covidethics.org/wp-content/uploads/2021/12/end-covax.pdf

[108] S Gundry. Abstract 10712: Observational findings of PULS cardiac test finding for inflammatory markers in patients receiving mRNA vaccines. Nov 8 2021. Circulation. 2021. 144: A10712. https://www.ahajournals.org/doi/10.1161/circ.144.suppl_1.10712

[109] C Huber. Heart damage from the COVID vaccines: Is it avoidable? Jul 14 2021. PDMJ. https://pdmj.org/papers/myocarditis_paper

[110] T Buzhdygan, B DeOre, et al. The SARS-CoV-2 spike protein alters barrier function in 2D static and 3D microfluidic in-vitro models of the human blood-brain barrier. Neurobiol Dis. Dec 2020. 146: 105131. https://www.ncbi.nlm.nih.gov/labs/pmc/articles/PMC7547916/

[111] J Schauer, S Buddhe, et al. Persistent cardiac MRI findings in a cohort of adolescents with post COVID-19 mRNA vaccine myopericarditis. J Pediatrics. Mar 25 2022. https://doi.org/10.1016/j.jpeds.2022.03.032

[112] S Seneff, G Nigh, et al. Innate immune suppression by SARS-CoV-2 mRNA vaccinations: the role of G-quadruplexes, exosomes and microRNAs. Jun 2022. Food and Chem Toxicol. 164: 113008. https://www.sciencedirect.com/science/article/pii/S027869152200206X?via%3Dihub

[113] F Fohse, B Geckin, et al. The BNT162b2 mRNA vaccine against SARS-CoV-2 reprograms both adaptive and innate immune responses. May 2021. MedRxiv. https://www.medrxiv.org/content/10.1101/2021.05.03.21256520v1.full-text

[114] Gov.UK Press Release: Government to provide shot in the arm for West Midlands vaccine manufacturing facility. Mar 31 2022. https://www.gov.uk/government/news/government-to-provide-shot-in-the-arm-for-west-midlands-vaccine-manufacturing-facility

[115] BioNTech. Securities and Exchange Commission Annual Report Form 20-F. Mar 30 2021. P. 28. https://investors.biontech.de/static-files/1b7360ae-c478-4d8f-bc7e-f0acc5316017

[116] S Reinfeld, R Cáceda, et al. Psychiatry Res. Oct 2021. 304. https://www.ncbi.nlm.nih.gov/pmc/articles/PMC8349391/

[117] Tedros Adhanom Ghebreyesus. World Health Organization. https://stevekirsch.substack.com/p/i-agree-with-who-dont-use-the-vaccines

[118] E Trigoso. 'What I've seen in the last 2 years is unprecedented': Physician on COVID vaccine side effects on pregnant women. Apr 27 2022. The Epoch Times. https://www.theepochtimes.com/what-ive-seen-in-the-last-two-years-is-unprecedented-physician-on-covid-vaccine-side-effects-on-pregnant-women_4428291.html

[119] Publishing Service.Gov.UK. COVID-19 mRNA Pfizer-BioNTech vaccine analysis print. P 81- 82. https://assets.publishing.service.gov.uk/government/uploads/system/uploads/attachment_data/file/1072043/COVID-19_mRNA_Pfizer-_BioNTech_vaccine_analysis_print.pdf

[120] S Suresh, Y Suzuki. SARS-CoV-2 spike protein and lung vascular cells. Dec 11 2020. J Respir 2021. 1 (1). 40-48. https://www.mdpi.com/2673-527X/1/1/4/htm

[121] Y Suzuki, S Gychka. SARS-CoV-2 spike protein elicits cell signaling in human host cells: implications for possible consequences of COVID-19 vaccines. Vaccines. Jan 2021. 9 (1): 36. https://www.ncbi.nlm.nih.gov/labs/pmc/articles/PMC7827936/

[122] S Zhang, Y Liu, et al. SARS-CoV-2 binds platelet ACE2 to enhance thrombosis in COVID-19. Sep 4 2020. J Hem Onc. https://jhoonline.biomedcentral.com/articles/10.1186/s13045-020-00954-7

[123] Canadian COVID Care Alliance. Hands off our children. Nov 6 2021. https://jhoonline.biomedcentral.com/articles/10.1186/s13045-020-00954-7

[124] C Huber. COVID-19 vaccine considerations. PrimaryDoctor. https://www.primarydoctor.org/covidvaccine

[125] S Gundry. Abstract 10712: Observational findings of PULS cardiac test finding for inflammatory markers in patients receiving mRNA vaccines. Nov 8 2021.

Circulation. 2021; 144: A10712.
https://www.ahajournals.org/doi/10.1161/circ.144.suppl_1.10712

[126] C Huber. Heart damage from the COVID vaccines: Is it avoidable? Jul 14 2021. PDMJ. https://pdmj.org/papers/myocarditis_paper

[127] S Seneff, G Nigh, et al. Innate immune suppression by SARS-CoV-2 mRNA vaccinations: the role of G-quadruplexes, exosomes and microRNAs. Jun 2022. Food and Chem Toxicol. 164: 113008.
https://www.sciencedirect.com/science/article/pii/S027869152200206X?via%3Dihub

[128] T Buzhdygan, B DeOre, et al. The SARS-CoV-2 spike protein alters barrier function in 2D static and 3D microfluidic in-vitro models of the human blood-brain barrier. Neurobiol Dis. Dec 2020. 146: 105131.
https://www.ncbi.nlm.nih.gov/labs/pmc/articles/PMC7547916/

[129] C Huber. Are the COVID vaccines bio-weapons? Aug 21 2021. The Defeat Of COVID. https://colleenhuber.substack.com/p/are-the-covid-vaccines-bio-weapons

[130] H Jiang, Y Mei. SARS-CoV-2 spike impairs DNA damage repair and inhibits V(D)J recombination in vitro. Aug 20 2021. Viruses. 13 (10) 2056.
https://www.mdpi.com/1999-4915/13/10/2056/htm?fbclid=IwAR1qAZFKzfHaIhN2Jjqfl1gMa4aJSoOTMs_JFk9iL6aysk5w-Zbz8BL0qHM

[131] P McCullough. Organ bio-distribution graph. Apr 10 2022. Twitter.

[132] Pfizer Confidential, obtained under Freedom of Information Act. SARS-CoV-2 mRNA vaccine. 2.6.4 Overview of pharmacokinetic test.
https://files.catbox.moe/0vwcmj.pdf

Chapter 3: Bradford Hill criteria for causality in health effects

[133] K Fedak, A Bernal, et al. Applying the Bradford Hill criteria in the 21st century: How data integration has changed causal inference in molecular epidemiology. Sep 30 2015. Emerg Themes Epidemiol.
https://www.ncbi.nlm.nih.gov/pmc/articles/PMC4589117/

[134] US Environmental Protection Agency. Memorandum. Nov 4 2015. https://www.epa.gov/sites/default/files/2015-11/documents/transmittal_of_final_redacted_report_to_mdeq.pdf

[135] University of Notre Dame. Virginia Tech researchers explain the Flint water crisis. Dec 8 2016. https://science.nd.edu/news/virginia-tech-researchers-explain-the-flint-water-crisis/#:~:text=The%20EPA%20recommends%20that%20water,was%20a%20staggering%2013%2C000%20ppb.

[136] J Dean. Water crisis took toll on Flint adults' physical, mental health. Apr 15 2021. Cornell Chronicle. https://news.cornell.edu/stories/2021/04/water-crisis-took-toll-flint-adults-physical-mental-health

[137] C Huber. Neither safe nor effective – The COVID vaccines are hazardous and should not be used. Apr 17 2022. https://colleenhuber.substack.com/p/neither-safe-nor-effective-the-covid?s=w

[138] J Smalley. COVID Requiem Aeternam. Apr 23 2022. https://metatron.substack.com/p/covid-requiem-aeternam

[139] Pfizer Worldwide Safety. 5.3.6 Cumulative analysis of post-authorization adverse event reports of PF-07302048 (BNT162B2) received through 28 Feb 2021. P 7. https://phmpt.org/wp-content/uploads/2021/11/5.3.6-postmarketing-experience.pdf

[140] US District Court. Northern District of Texas. Public Health and Medical Professionals for Transparency vs Food and Drug Administration. Sep 16 2021. Complaint for declaratory and injunctive relief. https://phmpt.org/wp-content/uploads/2021/10/001-Complaint-101021.pdf

[141] Centers for Disease Control and Prevention (CDC) Vaccine Adverse Event Reporting System (VAERS). https://wonder.cdc.gov/vaers.html

[142] Open VAERS. COVID vaccine data. https://openvaers.com/covid-data/mortality

[143] US Department of Health and Human Services. Vaccine Adverse Event Reporting System (VAERS). https://vaers.hhs.gov/

[144] US Centers for Disease Control and Prevention (CDC). https://wonder.cdc.gov/controller/datarequest/D8;jsessionid=B237772F95D48C57890B3BA7BBDF

[145] The Exposé. 12,548 children have suffered a serious adverse event due to the COVID vaccines in the USA; and 106 kids have sadly died. May 4 2022. The Exposé. https://dailyexpose.uk/2022/05/04/children-suffer-due-to-covid-vaccination/

[146] Pfizer BioNTech SE Confidential. Interim clinical study report – BNT 162-01 synopsis. Version 3.0. Mar 20 2021. P 12. https://phmpt.org/wp-content/uploads/2022/05/125742_S1_M5_5351_bnt162-01-interim3-synopsis.pdf

[147] J Rose. Silly adults, this one's for kids. May 9, 2022. Substack. https://jessicar.substack.com/p/silly-adults-this-ones-for-kids

[148] New York Times. Coronavirus in the US: Latest map and case count. Updated Apr 20 2022. https://www.nytimes.com/interactive/2021/us/covid-cases.html

[149] UK Health Security Agency. COVID-19 death rate per 100,000 individuals by vaccination status, Jan 3 to Mar 27 2022. The Exposé. https://dailyexpose.uk/2022/04/27/comparison-gov-reports-proves-vaccinated-suffering-ade/

[150] UK Publishing Service. COVID-19 mRNA Pfizer-BioNTech vaccine analysis print. Dec 9 2020 to Apr 20 2022. https://assets.publishing.service.gov.uk/government/uploads/system/uploads/attachment_data/file/1072043/COVID-19_mRNA_Pfizer-_BioNTech_vaccine_analysis_print.pdf

[151] A Dutt. Out of 34 Omicron cases at Delhi hospital, 33 are fully vaccinated. The Indian Express. Dec 23 2021. https://indianexpress.com/article/cities/delhi/out-of-34-omicron-cases-at-delhi-hospital-33-are-fully-vaccinated-7686188/

[152] Sen Ron Johnson. Video Release: Sen. Ron Johnson COVID-19 A Second Opinion Panel garners over 800,000 views in 24 hours. Jan 25 2022. https://www.ronjohnson.senate.gov/2022/1/video-release-sen-ron-johnson-covid-19-a-second-opinion-panel-garners-over-800-000-views-in-24-hours

[153] How much more evidence do you need? https://elcolectivodeuno.wordpress.com/2021/12/29/how-much-more-evidence-do-you-need-here-is-a-list-of-860-scientific-studies-and-reports-linking-covid-vaccines-to-hundreds-of-adverse-effects-and-deaths/

[154] The Exposé. Whilst you were distracted by Russia-Ukraine, the UK Gov revealed the triple-vaccinated seem to be developing acquired immunodeficiency syndrome. Apr 28 2022. The Exposé. https://dailyexpose.uk/2022/04/28/distracted-russia-gov-reveal-triple-jabbed-have-ai-ds/

[155] UK Health Security Agency. COVID-19 vaccine weekly surveillance reports (week 39 to 17, 2021 to 2022). https://www.gov.uk/government/publications/covid-19-vaccine-weekly-surveillance-reports

[156] UK Health Security Agency. COVID-19 vaccine surveillance report. Week 5. P. 47 https://assets.publishing.service.gov.uk/government/uploads/system/uploads/attachment_data/file/1052353/Vaccine_surveillance_report_-_week_5.pdf

[157] UK Health Security Agency. COVID-19 vaccine surveillance report. Week 9. P. 45. https://assets.publishing.service.gov.uk/government/uploads/system/uploads/attachment_data/file/1058464/Vaccine-surveillance-report-week-9.pdf

[158] UK Health Security Agency. COVID-19 vaccine surveillance report. Week 13. P. 45. https://assets.publishing.service.gov.uk/government/uploads/system/uploads/attachment_data/file/1066759/Vaccine-surveillance-report-week-13.pdf

[159] Pfizer Worldwide Safety. 5.3.6 Cumulative analysis of post-authorization adverse event reports of PF-07302048 (BNT162B2) received through 28-Feb-2021. Appendix 1: List of adverse events of special interest. https://phmpt.org/wp-content/uploads/2021/11/5.3.6-postmarketing-experience.pdf

[160] Siri Glimstad. Freedom of information Act Request to the Food and Drug Administration. Aug 27 2021. https://phmpt.org/wp-content/uploads/2021/10/IR0546-FDA-Pfizer-Approval-FINAL.pdf

[161] Aaron Siri. VDA produces the first 91+ pages of documents from Pfizer's COVID-19 vaccine file. Nov 19 2021. https://aaronsiri.substack.com/p/fda-produces-the-first-91-pages-of

[162] US Centers for Disease Control and Prevention (CDC) Myocarditis and Pericarditis. Nov 12 2021. https://www.cdc.gov/coronavirus/2019-ncov/vaccines/safety/myocarditis.html

[163] X Becerra. White House Convening on Equity. Apr 14 2022.
https://t.me/robinmg/18804

[164] J Horgan-Jones. The Irish Times. Jan 22 2022. Total of 100,000 Covid vaccines expire amid slowing demand, Ministers told.
https://www.irishtimes.com/news/ireland/irish-news/total-of-100-000-covid-vaccines-expire-amid-slowing-demand-ministers-told-1.4782708

[165] Johns Hopkins University. Our World in Data.
https://ourworldindata.org/coronavirus#explore-the-global-situation

[166] S Gazit, R Shlezinger, et al. SARS-CoV-2 naturally acquired immunity vs vaccine-induced immunity, reinfections vs breakthrough infections, a retrospective cohort study. Clin Infect Dis. Apr 5 2022.
https://academic.oup.com/cid/advance-article/doi/10.1093/cid/ciac262/6563799

[167] C Hansen, A Schelde, et al. Vaccine effectiveness against SARS-CoV-2 infection with the Omicron or Delta variants following a two-dose or booster BNT162b2 or mRNA-1273 vaccination series: A Danish cohort study.
https://www.medrxiv.org/content/10.1101/2021.12.20.21267966v3.full.pdf

[168] Status of the SARS-CoV-2 variant Omicron in Denmark. COVID-19 Omicron variant report. Dec 31 2021. Statens Serum Institut.
https://files.ssi.dk/covid19/omikron/statusrapport/rapport-omikronvarianten-31122021-ct18

[169] Karlstad, Hovi, et al. SARS-CoV-2 vaccination and myocarditis in a Nordic cohort study of 23 million residents. JAMA Cardiology. Apr 21 2022.
https://jamanetwork.com/journals/cardiology/articlepdf/2791253/jamacardiology_karlstad_2022_oi_220012_1649705559.15066.pdf

[170] US Department of Health and Human Services. Vaccine Adverse Event Reporting System (VAERS). https://vaers.hhs.gov/

[171] Open VAERS. COVID vaccine data. https://openvaers.com/covid-data/mortality

[172] J Rose. Silly adults, this one's for kids. May 9, 2022. Substack.
https://jessicar.substack.com/p/silly-adults-this-ones-for-kids

[173] L Sun, E Jaffe, et al. Increased emergency cardiovascular events among under-40 population in Israel during vaccine rollout and third COVID-19 wave. Apr 28 2022. Nature Scientific Reports. https://www.nature.com/articles/s41598-022-10928-z#Sec14

[174] Gov.UK. Information for healthcare professionals on COVID-19 vaccine Pfizer/BioNTech (Regulation 174): Myocarditis and pericarditis. Updated May 5 2022. https://www.gov.uk/government/publications/regulatory-approval-of-pfizer-biontech-vaccine-for-covid-19/information-for-healthcare-professionals-on-pfizerbiontech-covid-19-vaccine#efficacy

[175] A Chapman, A Shah, et al. Long-term outcomes in patients with type 2 myocardial infarction and myocardial injury. Circulation. Mar 20 2018. 137 (12). 1236-1245. https://www.ncbi.nlm.nih.gov/pmc/articles/PMC5882250/

[176] Office for National Statistics. Coronavirus (COVID-19) infection survey, UK: Characteristics related to having an Omicron compatible result in those who test positive for COVID-19. Dec 21 2021. https://www.ons.gov.uk/peoplepopulationandcommunity/healthandsocialcare/conditionsanddiseases/adhocs/14107coronaviruscovid19infectionsurveyukcharacteristicsrelatedtohavinganomicroncompatibleresultinthosewhotestpositiveforcovid19

[177] UK Health Security Agency. COVID-19 vaccine surveillance report. Week 9. Mar 3 2022. https://assets.publishing.service.gov.uk/government/uploads/system/uploads/attachment_data/file/1058464/Vaccine-surveillance-report-week-9.pdf

[178] UK Office for National Statistics. Deaths by vaccination status, England. https://www.ons.gov.uk/peoplepopulationandcommunity/birthsdeathsandmarriages/deaths/datasets/deathsbyvaccinationstatusengland

[179] Lifesite News. British children are up to 52 times more likely to die following a COVID shot. Feb 2 2022. https://www.lifesitenews.com/news/children-in-britain-up-to-52-times-more-likely-to-die-following-a-covid-shot-report-finds/

[180] UK Office for National Statistics. Age-standardised mortality rates by vaccination status, per 100,000 person-years, England, Age 10 to 14. Apr 27 2022 https://dailyexpose.uk/2022/04/27/kids-death-risk-increases-5100percent-covid-vaccination/

[181] R Steyer, G Kappler. The higher the vaccination rate, the higher the excess mortality. Nov 16 2021. https://www.skirsch.com/covid/GermanAnalysis.pdf

https://www.utebergner.de/cms/wp-content/uploads/2021/11/%C3%9Cbersterblichkeit-KW-36-bis-40-in-2021-003.docx

[182] Walgreens. Walgreens COVID-19 Index. Apr 3 2022 to Apr 19 2022. https://www.walgreens.com/businesssolutions/covid-19-index.jsp

[183] The Exposé. Official data suggests the Covid-19 injection is killing more people than it is saving. May 4 2022. https://dailyexpose.uk/2022/05/04/covid-vaccine-kills-more-than-it-saves/

[184] Government of Canada. COVID-19 daily epidemiology update. May 4 2022. https://health-infobase.canada.ca/covid-19/epidemiological-summary-covid-19-cases.html

[185] Karlstad, Hovi, et al. SARS-CoV-2 vaccination and myocarditis in a Nordic cohort study of 23 million residents. JAMA Cardiology. Apr 21 2022. https://jamanetwork.com/journals/cardiology/articlepdf/2791253/jamacardiology_karlstad_2022_oi_220012_1649705559.15066.pdf

[186] Gov.UK. Information for healthcare professionals on COVID-19 vaccine Pfizer/BioNTech (Regulation 174): Myocarditis and pericarditis. Updated May 5 2022. https://www.gov.uk/government/publications/regulatory-approval-of-pfizer-biontech-vaccine-for-covid-19/information-for-healthcare-professionals-on-pfizerbiontech-covid-19-vaccine#efficacy

[187] Moderna, Inc. Securities and Exchange Commission. Form 10-K Annual Report Feb 25 2022. P 59. https://investors.modernatx.com/financials/sec-filings/sec-filings-details/default.aspx?FilingId=15601998

[188] S Bhakdi, A Burkhardt. On COVID vaccines: Why they cannot work, and irrefutable evidence of their causative role in deaths after vaccination. https://doctors4covidethics.org/wp-content/uploads/2021/12/end-covax.pdf

[189] S Gundry. Abstract 10712: Observational findings of PULS cardiac test finding for inflammatory markers in patients receiving mRNA vaccines. Nov 8 2021. Circulation. 2021. 144: A10712. https://www.ahajournals.org/doi/10.1161/circ.144.suppl_1.10712

[190] C Huber. Heart damage from the COVID vaccines: Is it avoidable? Jul 14 2021. PDMJ. https://pdmj.org/papers/myocarditis_paper

[191] T Buzhdygan, B DeOre, et al. The SARS-CoV-2 spike protein alters barrier function in 2D static and 3D microfluidic in-vitro models of the human blood-brain barrier. Neurobiol Dis. Dec 2020. 146: 105131. https://www.ncbi.nlm.nih.gov/labs/pmc/articles/PMC7547916/

[192] L Malek, H Kaminska, et al. Children with acute myocarditis often have persistent subclinical changes as reviewed by cardiac magnetic resonance. J Magn Reson Imaging. 2020. 52: 488-496. https://pubmed.ncbi.nlm.nih.gov/31930765/

[193] S Dubey, A Agarwal, et al. Persistence of late gadolinium enhancement on follow-up CMR imaging in children with acute myocarditis. Dec 2020. Pediatr Cardiol. 41 (8). 1777-1782. https://pubmed.ncbi.nlm.nih.gov/32920654/

[194] J Schauer, S Buddhe, et al. Persistent cardiac MRI findings in a cohort of adolescents with post COVID-19 mRNA vaccine myopericarditis. J Pediatrics. Mar 25 2022. https://doi.org/10.1016/j.jpeds.2022.03.032

[195] F Fohse, B Geckin, et al. The BNT162b2 mRNA vaccine against SARS-CoV-2 reprograms both adaptive and innate immune responses. May 2021. MedRxiv. https://www.medrxiv.org/content/10.1101/2021.05.03.21256520v1.full-text

[196] S Seneff, G Nigh, et al. Innate immune suppression by SARS-CoV-2 mRNA vaccinations: the role of G-quadruplexes, exosomes and microRNAs. Jun 2022. Food and Chem Toxicol. 164: 113008. https://www.sciencedirect.com/science/article/pii/S027869152200206X?via%3Dihub

[197] D Follmann, H Janes, et al. Anti-nucleocapsid antibodies following SARS-CoV-2 infection in the blinded phase of the mRNA-1273 Covid-19 vaccine efficacy clinical trial. Apr 19 2022. medRxiv. https://www.medrxiv.org/content/10.1101/2022.04.18.22271936v1

[198] W Lee, A Wheatley, et al. Antibody-dependent enhancement and SARS-CoV-2 vaccines and therapies. Sep 9 2020. Nature Microbiology. https://www.nature.com/articles/s41564-020-00789-5

[199] S Kirsch, J Rose, M Crawford. Estimating the number of COVID vaccine deaths in America. Dec 24 2021. https://www.skirsch.com/covid/Deaths.pdf

[200] S Kirsch. Latest VAERS estimate: 388,000 Americans killed by the COVID vaccines. Dec 14 2021. Steve Kirsch's Newsletter. https://stevekirsch.substack.com/p/latest-vaers-estimate-388000-americans

[201] Public Health Scotland. Public Health Scotland COVID-19 & Winter Statistical Report. Jan 17 2022. https://publichealthscotland.scot/media/11802/22-01-19-covid19-winter_publication_report_revised.pdf

[202] J Murphy, C Huber. Student athletes perform worse than controls following COVID vaccines. Jan 16 2022. PDMJ. https://pdmj.org/papers/Student_athletes_perform_worse_than_controls_foll owing_COVID_vaccines

[203] Real Science. 942 athlete cardiac arrests, serious issues, 621 dead, after COVID shot. https://goodsciencing.com/covid/athletes-suffer-cardiac-arrest-die-after-covid-shot/

[204] S Zhang, Y Xu, et al. Cationic compounds used in lipoplexes and polyplexes for gene delivery. Nov 24 2004. J Controlled Release. https://www.sciencedirect.com/science/article/abs/pii/S0168365904004006?v ia%3Dihub

[205] S Ndeupen, Z Qin, et al. The mRNA-LNP platform's lipid nanoparticle component used in preclinical vaccine studies is highly inflammatory. Nov 19 2021. CellPress. https://www.cell.com/action/showPdf?pii=S2589-0042%2821%2901450-4

[206] C Tseng, E Sbrana. Immunization with SARS coronavirus vaccines leads to pulmonary immunopathology on challenge with the SARS virus. Apr 20 2012. PLoS One. https://www.ncbi.nlm.nih.gov/pmc/articles/PMC3335060/

[207] H Weingarti, M Czub, et al. Immunization with modified vaccinia virus Ankara-based recombinant vaccine against severe acute respiratory syndrome is associated with enhanced hepatitis in ferrets. Nov 2004. J Virol. https://www.ncbi.nlm.nih.gov/pmc/articles/PMC525089/

[208] How much more evidence do you need? https://elcolectivodeuno.wordpress.com/2021/12/29/how-much-more-evidence-do-you-need-here-is-a-list-of-860-scientific-studies-and-reports-linking-covid-vaccines-to-hundreds-of-adverse-effects-and-deaths/

Chapter 4: Secondary vaccine effects

[209] American Society of Clinical Oncology (ASCO). Cancer.net. Understanding radiation therapy. https://www.cancer.net/navigating-cancer-care/how-cancer-treated/radiation-therapy/understanding-radiation-therapy#:~:text=Permanent%20implants%20remain%20radioactive%20after,with%20children%20or%20pregnant%20women

[210] Cancer Research UK. Internal radiotherapy safety. https://www.cancerresearchuk.org/about-cancer/cancer-in-general/treatment/radiotherapy/internal/safety

[211] VAERS Vaccine Adverse Event Reporting System, VAERS Data. https://vaers.hhs.gov/data.html

[212] Aaron Siri. VDA produces the first 91+ pages of documents from Pfizer's COVID-19 vaccine file. Nov 19 2021. https://aaronsiri.substack.com/p/fda-produces-the-first-91-pages-of

[213] Siri Glimstad. Freedom of information Act Request to the Food and Drug Administration. Aug 27 2021. https://phmpt.org/wp-content/uploads/2021/10/IR0546-FDA-Pfizer-Approval-FINAL.pdf

[214] Pfizer Worldwide Safety. 5.3.6 Cumulative analysis of post-authorization adverse event reports of PF-07302048 (BNT162B2) received through 28-Feb-2021. Appendix 1: List of adverse events of special interest. https://phmpt.org/wp-content/uploads/2021/11/5.3.6-postmarketing-experience.pdf

[215] Naomi Wolf PhD had begun to gather informal reports from individuals on social media regarding menstrual irregularities in family members of recently vaccinated people. Before that information was consolidated or analyzed, she was suspended from Twitter. This BBC article is too biased to attain credibility, but gives the key event of discussion of vaccine secondary effects and the June 5-6, 2021 timeframe of Wolf's suspension from Twitter, which is close in time to peak incidence of secondary effects in this study.

https://www.bbc.com/news/world-us-canada-57374241 None of the prominent MSM smear articles on the event of Wolf's suspension from Twitter reveal any attempt to interview Wolf, and one of her detractors claims that he "took an hour on the internet" to refute her, leaving the reader without confidence in the veracity of such articles.
https://www.businessinsider.com/whos-afraid-of-naomi-wolf-2021-6 It is possible that the empirical data that Wolf had begun to gather may be lost permanently.

[216] Pfizer. A Phase 1/2/3, placebo-controlled, randomized, observer-blind, dose-finding study to evaluate the safety, tolerability, immunogenicity, and efficacy of SARS-CoV-2 RNA vaccine candidates against COVID-19 in healthy individuals. Pp. 67-68. https://cdn.pfizer.com/pfizercom/2020-11/C4591001_Clinical_Protocol_Nov2020.pdf

[217] R Kedl, E Hsieh, et al. Evidence for aerosol transfer of SARS-CoV-2 -specific humoral immunity. May 1 2022. medRxiv.
https://www.medrxiv.org/content/10.1101/2022.04.28.22274443v1.full-text

[218] B Ventura, et al. Toxicity of spike fragments of SARS-CoV-2 S protein for zebrafish: A tool to study its hazards for human health. Sci Total Environ. Mar 20 2022. https://pubmed.ncbi.nlm.nih.gov/34942250/

Chapter 5: Student athletes

[219] COVID-19 vaccines: scientific proof of lethality. Jan 5 2022.
https://www.saveusnow.org.uk/covid-vaccine-scientific-proof-lethal/

[220] Pfizer Worldwide Safety. Cumulative analysis of post-authorization adverse event reports of PF-07302048 (BNT162B2) received through 28-Feb-2021.
https://phmpt.org/wp-content/uploads/2021/11/5.3.6-postmarketing-experience.pdf.
Pp. 30-38.

[221] US District Court. Northern District of Texas. Public Health and Medical Professionals for Transparency v Food and Drug Administration. Complaint for declaratory and injunctive relief. https://phmpt.org/wp-content/uploads/2021/10/001-Complaint-101021.pdf

[222] S Bhakdi, A Burkhardt. On COVID vaccines: why they cannot work, and irrefutable evidence of their causative role in deaths after vaccination. https://doctors4covidethics.org/wp-content/uploads/2021/12/end-covax.pdf

[223] S Gundry. Abstract 10712: Observational findings of PULS cardiac test finding for inflammatory markers in patients receiving mRNA vaccines. Circulation. Nov 8 2021. https://www.ahajournals.org/doi/abs/10.1161/circ.144.suppl_1.10712

[224] Ibid.

[225] C Huber. Heart damage from the COVID vaccines: Is it avoidable? PDMJ 3. Jul 14 2021. https://pdmj.org/papers/myocarditis_paper

Chapter 6: Heart damage

[226] US Centers for Disease Control (CDC). Clinical considerations: Myocarditis and pericarditis after receipt of mRNA COVID-19 vaccines among adolescents and young adults. May 28 2021. https://www.cdc.gov/vaccines/covid-19/clinical-considerations/myocarditis.html

[227] S Mouch, A Roguin, et al. Myocarditis following COVID-19 mRNA vaccination. Jun 29 2021. Vaccine. 39 (29). 3790-3793. https://www.ncbi.nlm.nih.gov/pmc/articles/PMC8162819/

[228] J Su, M McNeil, et al. Myopericarditis after vaccination, Vaccine Adverse Event Reporting System (VAERS), 1990-2018. Jan 29 2021. Vaccine. 39 (5): 839-845. https://pubmed.ncbi.nlm.nih.gov/33422381/

[229] A Lala, K Johnson, et al. Prevalence and impact of myocardial injury in patients hospitalized with COVID-19 infection. Aug 4 2020. J Am Coll Cardiol. 76 (5). 533-546. https://www.ncbi.nlm.nih.gov/pmc/articles/PMC7279721/

[230] A Chapman, A Shah, et al. Long-term outcomes in patients with type 2 myocardial infarction and myocardial injury. Mar 20 2018. Circulation. 137 (12). 1236-1245. https://www.ncbi.nlm.nih.gov/pmc/articles/PMC5882250/

[231] H Yamakawa, M Ieda. Cardiac regeneration by direct reprogramming in this decade and beyond. Jul 1 2021. Inflamm Regen. 41 (20). https://www.ncbi.nlm.nih.gov/pmc/articles/PMC8247073/

[232] R Hodkinson MD, interviewed on The High Wire by Del Bigtree, Episode 220. Jun 17 2021. https://thehighwire.com/watch/

[233] P McCullough. A cardiologist's view of long-haul syndrome and COVID-19 vaccine injury: A path forward for clinicians. Apr 10 2022. Environmental Health Symposium. Tucson. AZ https://www.environmentalhealthsymposium.com/schedule-2022

[234] P McCullough. Twitter. https://twitter.com/p-mcculloughmd/status/1513731434992656390

[235] S Mouch, A Roguin, et al. Myocarditis following COVID-19 mRNA vaccination. Jun 29 2021. Vaccine. 39 (29). 3790-3793. https://www.ncbi.nlm.nih.gov/pmc/articles/PMC8162819/

[236] M Polito, A Silverio, et al. Cardiovascular involvement in COVID-19: What sequelae should we expect? Jun 30 2021. Cardiol Ther. 1-20. https://www.ncbi.nlm.nih.gov/pmc/articles/PMC8243311/#CR4

[237] C Huber. Lockdowns failed to reduce deaths in the US. Jun 12, 2020. PDMJ. https://pdmj.org/papers/lockdowns_failed_to_reduce_deaths_in_the_us/

[238] Our World in Data. Coronavirus (COVID-19) vaccinations. Jul 10 2021. https://ourworldindata.org/covid-vaccinations

[239] United Nations, Dept of Economic and Social Affairs, World population prospects. World death rate, 1950-2021. https://www.macrotrends.net/countries/WLD/world/death-rate

[240] 'We made a big mistake' – COVID vaccine spike protein travels from injection site, can cause organ damage. June 3 2021. The Defender. https://childrenshealthdefense.org/defender/covid-vaccine-spike-protein-travels-from-injection-site-organ-damage/

[241] SARS-CoV-2 mRNA vaccine. Pfizer report, Japanese government. [Document in both Japanese and English] p.7 of the English section. https://www.docdroid.net/xq0Z8B0/pfizer-report-japanese-government-pdf

[242] M Polito, A Silverio, et al. Cardiovascular involvement in COVID-19: What sequelae should we expect? Jun 30 2021. Cardiol Ther. 1-20. https://www.ncbi.nlm.nih.gov/pmc/articles/PMC8243311/#CR4

[243] A Karamyshev, Z Karamysheva. Lost in translation: Ribosome-associated mRNA and protein quality controls. Oct 4 2018 Front. Genet. . https://www.frontiersin.org/articles/10.3389/fgene.2018.00431/full

[244] S Ravinidis, E Doxakis. RNA-binding proteins implicated in mitochondrial damage and mitophagy. 2020. Front Cell Dev Biol. 8 (372). https://www.ncbi.nlm.nih.gov/pmc/articles/PMC7287033/

[245] R Kawakami, A Sakamoto. Pathological evidence for SARS-CoV-2 as a cause of myocarditis. Jan 26 2021. J Am Coll Cardiol. 77 (3). 314-325. https://www.ncbi.nlm.nih.gov/pmc/articles/PMC7816957/

[246] T Kotecha, D Knight, et al. Patterns of myocardial injury in recovered troponin-positive COVID-19 patients assessed by cardiovascular magnetic resonance. May 14 2021. Eur Heart J. 42 (19). 1866-1878. https://www.ncbi.nlm.nih.gov/pmc/articles/PMC7928984/

[247] D Bojkova, J Wagner, et al. SARS-CoV-2 infects and induces cytotoxic effects in human cardiomyocytes. Dec 1 2020. Cardiovasc Res. 116 (14): 2207-2215. https://pubmed.ncbi.nlm.nih.gov/32966582/

[248] G Tavazzi, C Pellegrini, et al. Myocardial localization of coronavirus in COVID-19 cardiogenic shock. Apr 10 2020. Eur J Heart Failure. https://onlinelibrary.wiley.com/doi/10.1002/ejhf.1828

[249] S Sala, G Peretto, et al. Acute myocarditis presenting as a reverse Tako-Tsubo syndrome in a patient with SARS-CoV-2 respiratory infection. May 14 2020. Eur Heart J. 41 (9). 1861-1862. https://academic.oup.com/eurheartj/article/41/19/1861/5817735

[250] M Imazio, K Klingel, et al. COVID-19 pandemic and troponin: indirect myocardial injury, myocardial inflammation or myocarditis? Aug 2020. Heart. 106 (15). 1127-1131. https://heart.bmj.com/content/106/15/1127

[251] M Imazio, K Klingel, et al. Ibid.

[252] A Wrobel, D Benton, et al. SARS-CoV-2 and bat RaTG13 spike glycoprotein structures inform on virus evolution and furin cleavage effects. Aug 1 2020. Nat Struct Mol Biol. 27(8). 763-767. https://www.ncbi.nlm.nih.gov/pmc/articles/PMC7610980/

[253] T Buzhdygan, B DeOre, et al. The SARS-CoV-2 spike protein alters barrier function in 2D static and 3D microfluidic in-vitro models of the human blood-

brain barrier. Dec 2020. Neurobiol Dis. 146: 105131.
https://www.ncbi.nlm.nih.gov/pmc/articles/PMC7547916/

[254] M Hoffman, H Kleine-Weber, et al. SARS-CoV-2 cell entry depends on ACE2 and TMPRSS2 and is blocked by a clinically proven protease inhibitor. Apr 16 2020. Cell. 181(2): 271-280.
https://www.ncbi.nlm.nih.gov/pmc/articles/PMC7102627/

[255] F Polack, S Thomas, et al. Safety and efficacy of the BNT162b2 mRNA COVID-19 vaccine. Dec 10 2020. N Engl J Med.
https://www.ncbi.nlm.nih.gov/pmc/articles/PMC7745181/

[256] A Choudhury, N Das, et al. Exploring the binding efficacy of ivermectin against the key proteins of SARS-CoV-2 pathogenesis: an in silico approach. Mar 25 2021. Future Vir. https://www.futuremedicine.com/doi/10.2217/fvl-2020-0342

[257] COVID-19 early treatment: real-time analysis of 724 studies.
https://c19early.com/

[258] H Zhang, J Penninger, et al. Angiotensin-converting enzyme 2 (ACE2) as a SARS-CoV-2 receptor: molecular mechanisms and potential therapeutic target. 2020. Intensive Care Med. 46 (4). 586-590.
https://www.ncbi.nlm.nih.gov/pmc/articles/PMC7079879/

[259] L Chen, X Li, et al. The ACE2 expression in human heart indicates new potential mechanism of heart injury among patients infected with SARS-CoV-2. Mar 30 2020. Cardiovasc Res.
https://www.ncbi.nlm.nih.gov/pmc/articles/PMC7184507/

[260] A Goulter, M Goddard, et al. ACE2 gene expression is up-regulated in the human failing heart. May 19 2004. BMC Med. 2 (19).
https://www.ncbi.nlm.nih.gov/pmc/articles/PMC425604/

[261] Y Lei, J Zhang, et al. SARS-CoV-2 spike protein impairs endothelial function via downregulation of ACE 2. Mar 31 2021. Circulation Res. 128 (9).
https://www.ahajournals.org/doi/10.1161/CIRCRESAHA.121.318902

[262] Y Lei, J Zhang, et al. Ibid.

[263] K Wang, W Chen, et al. CD147-spike protein is a novel route for SARS-CoV-2 infection to host cells. 2020. Signal Transduct Target Ther. 5. 283.
https://www.ncbi.nlm.nih.gov/pmc/articles/PMC7714896/

[264] D Bojkova, J Wagner, et al. SARS-CoV-2 infects and induces cytotoxic effects in human cardiomyocytes. Dec 1 2020. Cardiovasc Res. 116 (14): 2207-2215. https://pubmed.ncbi.nlm.nih.gov/32966582/

[265] Y Lei, J Zhang, et al. SARS-CoV-2 spike protein impairs endothelial function via downregulation of ACE 2. Mar 31 2021. Circulation Res. 128 (9). https://www.ahajournals.org/doi/10.1161/CIRCRESAHA.121.318902

[266] E Avolio, M Gamez, et al. The SARS-CoV-2 spike protein disrupts the cooperative function of human cardiac pericytes – endothelial cells through CD 147 receptor-mediated signaling: a potential non-infective mechanism of COVID-19 microvascular disease. Dec 21 2020. bioRxiv. https://www.biorxiv.org/content/10.1101/2020.12.21.423721v1.full

[267] Y Lei, J Zhang, et al. SARS-CoV-2 spike protein impairs endothelial function via downregulation of ACE 2. Mar 31 2021. Circulation Res. 128 (9). https://www.ahajournals.org/doi/10.1161/CIRCRESAHA.121.318902

[268] S Hojyo, M Uchida, et al. How COVID-19 induces cytokine storm with high mortality. Oct 1 2020. Europe PMC. .40:37. https://europepmc.org/article/PMC/PMC7527296

[269] G Torre-Amione, S Kapadia, et al. Proinflammatory cytokine levels in patients with depressed left ventricular ejection fraction. 1996. J Am Coll Card. 27. 1201-1206. https://www.sciencedirect.com/science/article/pii/0735109795005897?via%3Dihub

[270] E Avolio, M Gamez, et al. The SARS-CoV-2 spike protein disrupts the cooperative function of human cardiac pericytes – endothelial cells through CD 147 receptor-mediated signaling: a potential non-infective mechanism of COVID-19 microvascular disease. Dec 21 2020. bioRxiv. https://www.biorxiv.org/content/10.1101/2020.12.21.423721v1.full

[271] S Mouch, A Roguin, et al. Myocarditis following COVID-19 mRNA vaccination. Jun 29 2021. Vaccine. 39 (29). 3790-3793. https://www.ncbi.nlm.nih.gov/pmc/articles/PMC8162819/

[272] P McCullough. May 1 2022. Twitter. https://twitter.com/p_mcculloughmd/status/1520731761818415104

[273] B Brouha, J Schustak, et al. Hot L1s account for the bulk of retrotransposition in the human population. Apr 29 2003. Proc Natl Acad Sci USA, 100 (9). 5280-5285. https://www.ncbi.nlm.nih.gov/pmc/articles/PMC154336/

[274] L Zhang, A Richards, et al. Reverse-transcribed SARS-CoV-2 RNA can integrate into the genome of cultured human cells and can be expressed in patient-derived tissues. May 6 2021. PNAS. https://www.pnas.org/doi/10.1073/pnas.2105968118

[275] H Jiang, Y Mei. SARS-CoV-2 spike impairs DNA damage repair and inhibits V(D)J recombination in vitro. 2021. Viruses. 13 (10). 2056. https://www.mdpi.com/1999-4915/13/10/2056

[276] M Aldén, F Falla, et al. Intracellular reverse transcription of Pfizer BioNTech COVID-19 mRNA vaccine BNT162b2 in vitro in human liver cell line. Feb 23 2022. MDPI. https://www.mdpi.com/1467-3045/44/3/73/htm

Chapter 7: Fluid dynamics

[277] F Angeli, A Spanevello, et al. SARS-CoV-2 vaccines: Lights and shadows. Jun 1 2021. Eur J Int Med. Vol 88. P1-8. https://www.ejinme.com/article/S0953-6205(21)00142-4/fulltext

[278] M Deshotels, H Xia, et al. Angiotensin II mediates angiotensin converting enzyme type 2 internalization and degradation through an angiotensin II type I receptor-dependent mechanism. Dec 2014. Hypertension. 64 (6): 1368-1375. https://pubmed.ncbi.nlm.nih.gov/25225202/

[279] S Zhang, Y Liu et al. SARS-CoV-2 binds platelet ACE2 to enhance thrombosis in COVID-19. Sep 4 2020. J Hematol Oncol. 13 (1): 120. https://pubmed.ncbi.nlm.nih.gov/32887634/

[280] C Huber. Heart damage from the COVID vaccines: Is it avoidable? Jul 14 2021. PDMJ. https://pdmj.org/papers/myocarditis_paper

[281] Z Strieber. Heart inflammation more prevalent among vaccinated than unvaccinated: study. Apr 22 2022. The Epoch Times. https://www.theepochtimes.com/heart-inflammation-higher-among-vaccinated-than-unvaccinated-study_4420652.html

[282] P McCullough. May 1 2022. Twitter.
https://twitter.com/p_mcculloughmd/status/1520731761818415104

Chapter 8: What is in a vaccine?

[283] B Pulendran, P Arunachalam, D O'Hagan. Emerging concepts in the science of vaccine adjuvants. Apr 6 2021. Nat Rev Drug Discov. 1-22.
https://www.ncbi.nlm.nih.gov/pmc/articles/PMC8023785/

[284] Oxford Materials Safety Data Sheets.
https://www.oxfordasd.org/domain/1183

[285] D Zhu, W Tuo. QS-21: A potent vaccine adjuvant. Apr 2016. Nat Prod Chem Res. 3 (4): e113. https://www.ncbi.nlm.nih.gov/pmc/articles/PMC4874334/

[286] M Picard, J Drolet, et al. Safety of COVID-19 vaccination in patients with polyethylene glycol allergy: A case series. Dec 20 2021. J Allergy Clin Immunol Pract. 10 (2): 6620-625.
https://www.ncbi.nlm.nih.gov/pmc/articles/PMC8685412/

[287] Oxford Materials Safety Data Sheets.
https://www.oxfordasd.org/domain/1183

[288] K Wylon, S Dölle, M Worm. Polyethylene glycol as a cause of anaphylaxis. Dec 13 2016. Allergy, Asthma & Clin Immun. 12 (67).
https://aacijournal.biomedcentral.com/articles/10.1186/s13223-016-0172-7

[289] S Zhang, Y Xu, et al. Cationic compounds used in lipoplexes and polyplexes for gene delivery. Nov 24 2004. J Controlled Release. 100 (2). 165 – 180.
https://www.sciencedirect.com/science/article/abs/pii/S0168365904004006?via%3Dihub

[290] C Huber. Are the COVID vaccines bio-weapons? Aug 21 2021. Substack.
https://colleenhuber.substack.com/p/are-the-covid-vaccines-bio-weapons

[291] CDC. FAQs vaccination for children & teens.
https://www.cdc.gov/coronavirus/2019-ncov/vaccines/faq-children.html

[292] Oxford Materials Safety Data Sheets.
https://www.oxfordasd.org/domain/1183

[293] W Thomas. Supreme Court Review of the OSHA benzene standard. 36 (3) Part 2. Taylor & Francis. https://www.jstor.org/stable/2683839

[294] US Code of Federal Regulations. 45 CFR § 46.116 (b) (8). Title 45: Public Welfare. Subtitle A: Department of Health and Human Serives. Subchapter A: General Administration. Part 46: Protection of Human Subjects. Reprinted in Legal Information Institute, Cornell Law School. https://www.law.cornell.edu/cfr/text/45/46.116

[295] D Horowitz. Horowitz: Why there is an urgent need to study effects of COVID shots on reproductive health. May 3 2022. Conservative Review. https://www.conservativereview.com/horowitz-why-there-is-an-urgent-need-to-study-effects-of-covid-shots-on-reproductive-health-2657257803.html

[296] FDA. Summary basis for regulatory action. Nov 8 2021. https://www.fda.gov/media/151733/download

[297] C Klaasen. Casarett & Doull's Toxicology: The Basic Science of Poisons. 8th ed. McGraw Hill. 2013.

Chapter 9: Immunology 101.1

[298] A Fauci. Interview with the Washington Journal. Oct 11 2004. C-SPAN. https://twitter.com/p_mcculloughmd/status/1511898738494738433?s=21&t=UqRVE9grUVF8JMS5a_D76w

[299] Blood. Miltenyi Biotec. https://www.miltenyibiotec.com/US-en/resources/macs-handbook/human-cells-and-organs/human-cell-sources/blood-human.html

[300] R Akonda, M Fitch, et al. Origin and differentiation of human memory CD8 T cells after vaccination. Dec 2017. Nature. 552 (7685). https://pid.emory.edu/ark:/25593/t3gvx

[301] S Duffy. Why are RNA virus mutation rates so damn high? Aug 2018. PLoS Biologyhttps://journals.plos.org/plosbiology/article?id=10.1371/journal.pbio.3000003

Chapter 10: Would you buy a used car from these companies?

302 A Clark. Pfizer drug breach ends in biggest US crime fine. Sep 2 2009. The Guardian. https://www.theguardian.com/business/2009/sep/02/pfizer-drugs-us-criminal-fine

303 L Girion. Johnson & Johnson knew for decades that asbestos lurked in its baby powder. Dec 14 2018. Reuters Investigates. https://www.reuters.com/investigates/special-report/johnsonandjohnson-cancer/

304 N Kresge and Bloomberg. Moderna has never distributed a product before. A Swiss company is here to help. Nov 19 2020. Fortune. https://fortune.com/2020/11/19/moderna-vaccine-distribution-lonza-swiss/

305 I Chudov. Moderna patented cancer gene is in SARS-CoV-2 "spike protein." Feb 22 2022. https://igorchudov.substack.com/p/moderna-patented-cancer-gene-is-in

306 United States Patent. Bancel et al. Patent No: US 9,587,003 B2. Mar 7 2017. https://patentimages.storage.googleapis.com/01/6e/60/8951ab8f4118b5/US9587003.pdf

307 M Wallace. Moderna CEO admits it's possible that the vaccine maker patented DNA three years before the pandemic could match genetic [sic] in the COVID-19 virus. Feb 2022. https://dcweekly.org/2022/03/02/moderna-ceo-admits-its-possible-that-the-vaccine-maker-patented-dna-three-years-before-the-pandemic-could-match-genetic-in-the-covid-19-virus/

308 C Huber. The Defeat Of COVID. Apr 2021. https://www.amazon.com/Defeat-COVID-medical-studies-doesnt-ebook/dp/B0926RX9J1/ref=sr_1_1

309 Associated Press. Denmark to destroy excess soon-to-expire COVID-19 vaccines. May 2 2022. ABC News. https://abcnews.go.com/Health/wireStory/denmark-destroy-excess-expire-covid-19-vaccines-84441932

Chapter 11: Vitamin D vs vaccines

[310] C Tseng, E Sbrana, et al. Immunization with SARS Coronavirus vaccines leads to pulmonary immunopathology on challenge with the SARS virus. Apr 20 2012. PLoS One. 7 (4). https://www.ncbi.nlm.nih.gov/pmc/articles/PMC3335060/

[311] M Zhang, J Sun, et al. Modified mRNA-LNP vaccines confer protection against experimental DENV-2 infection in mice. Sep 11 2020. Mol Therapy Methods & Clin Dev. 18: 702-712. https://www.sciencedirect.com/science/article/pii/S2329050120301625

[312] F Arkin. Dengue vaccine fiasco leads to criminal charges for researcher in the Philippines. Apr 24 2019. Science. https://www.science.org/content/article/dengue-vaccine-fiasco-leads-criminal-charges-researcher-philippines

[313] B Bridle. Coronavirus vaccine concerns: "I would prefer to have natural immunity." Feb 24 2021. Dryburgh.com. https://dryburgh.com/byram-bridle-coronavirus-vaccine-concerns/

[314] C Huber. Trading COVID for heart disease buys you both. Jan 11 2022. Substack. https://colleenhuber.substack.com/p/trading-covid-for-heart-disease-buys

[315] S Manolagas, D Provvedini, et al. Interactions of 1,25-dihydroxyvitamin D3 and the immune system. Dec 1985. Mol Cell Endocrinol. 43 (2-3). 113-22. https://pubmed.ncbi.nlm.nih.gov/3000847/

[316] X Yu, H Mocharla, et al. Vitamin D receptor expression in human lymphocytes. Signal requirements and characterization by western blots and DNA sequencing. Apr 25 1991. J Biol Chem. 266 (12). 7588-95. https://pubmed.ncbi.nlm.nih.gov/1850412/

[317] R Wiese, A Uhland-Smith, et al. Up-regulation of the vitamin D receptor in response to 1,25-dihydroxyvitamin D3 results from ligand-induced stabilization. Oct 5 1992. J Biol Chem. 267. 20082-20086. https://pubmed.ncbi.nlm.nih.gov/1328192/

[318] M Cantorna. Mechanisms underlying the effect of vitamin D on the immune system. Jun 2 2010. Cambridge Univ Press. https://www.cambridge.org/core/journals/proceedings-of-the-nutrition-society/article/mechanisms-underlying-the-effect-of-vitamin-d-on-the-immune-system/91FB1F56494E909053590AE99E4C6DC4

[319] J Lemire, D Archer, et al. Immmunosuppressive actions of 1,25-dihydroxyvitamin D3: preferential inhibition of TH1 functions. Jun 1995. J Nutr 125 (6 Suppl). 1704S-1708S. https://academic.oup.com/jn/article-abstract/125/suppl_6/1704S/4730957?redirectedFrom=fulltext

[320] I Alroy, T Towers, et al. Transcriptional repression of the interleukin-2 gene by vitamin D3: Direct inhibition of NFAT//AP-1 complex formation by a nuclear hormone receptor. Oct 1 1995. Am Soc Microbio J. https://mcb.asm.org/content/15/10/5789

[321] J Adams, M Hewison. Unexpected actions of vitamin D: new perspectives on the regulation of innate and adaptive immunity. Jan 31 2008. Nat Clin Pract Endocrinol Metab. 4 (2). 80-90. https://europepmc.org/article/PMC/2678245

[322] M Hewison. An update on vitamin D and human immunity. Feb 29 2012. Clin Endocrinol (Oxf). 76 (3). 315-325. https://europepmc.org/article/MED/21995874

[323] F Baeke, H Korf, et al. The vitamin D analog TX527, promotes a human CD4, CD25 high, CD127 low regulatory T cell profile and induces a migratory signature specific for homing to sites of inflammation. Jan 1 2011. J Immunol. 186 (1). 132-142. https://www.jimmunol.org/content/186/1/132.long

[324] M Kongsbak, T Levring, et al. The vitamin D receptor and T cell function. Jun 18 2013. Front Immunol. https://www.frontiersin.org/articles/10.3389/fimmu.2013.00148/full#B8

[325] S Hansdottir, M Monick, et al. Respiratory epithelial cells convert inactive vitamin D to its active form: potential effects on host defense. Oct 31 2008. J Immunol 181. (10). 7090 – 7099. https://europepmc.org/article/PMC/2596683

[326] P Smith, G Lombardi, et al. Type I interferons and the innate immune response-more than just antiviral cytokines. Jan 12 2005. Mol Immunol. 42 (8). 869-877. https://europepmc.org/article/MED/15829276

[327] J Hiscott. Triggering the innate antiviral response through IRF-3 activation. Mar 28 2007. J Biol Chem. 282 (21). 15325-15329. https://europepmc.org/article/MED/17395583

[328] A Stoppelenburg, J von Hegedus, et al. Defective control of vitamin D receptor-mediated epithelial STAT1 signalling predisposes to severe respiratory syncytial virus bronchiolitis. Sep 19 2013. J Path. 232 (1). 57-64. https://onlinelibrary.wiley.com/doi/abs/10.1002/path.4267

[329] A Hornsleth, L Loland, et al. Cytokines and chemokines in respiratory secretion and severity of disease in infants with respiratory syncytial virus (RSV) infection. Apr 30 2001. J Clin Virol. 21 (2). 163-170. https://europepmc.org/article/MED/11378497

[330] J Van Woensel and J Kimpen. Therapy for respiratory tract infections caused by respiratory syncytial virus. May 31 2000. Eur J Ped. 159 (6). 391-398. https://europepmc.org/article/MED/10867842

[331] S Hansdottir, M Monick, et al. Vitamin D decreases respiratory syncytial virus induction of NF-kappa-B-linked chemokines and cytokines in airway epithelium while maintaining the antiviral state. Dec 10 2009. J Immunol. 184 (2). 965-974. https://europepmc.org/article/PMC/3035054#R80

[332] E Villamor. A potential role for vitamin D on HIV infection? May 2006. Nutr Rev. 64 (5). 226-233. https://academic.oup.com/nutritionreviews/article/64/5/226/1910640

[333] R Connor, W Rigby. 1 alpha, 25-dihydroxyvitamin D3 inhibits productive infection of human monocytes by HIV-1. Mar 31 1991. Biochem Biophys Res Comm. 176 (2). 852-859. https://www.sciencedirect.com/science/article/abs/pii/S0006291X05802645?via%3Dihub

[334] A Braun, D Chang, et al. Association of low serum 25-hydroxyvitamin D levels and mortality in the critically ill. Mar 31 2011. Crit Care Med. 39 (4). 671-677. https://europepmc.org/article/PMC/3448785

[335] L Mathews, Y Ahmed, et al. Worsening severity of vitamin D deficiency is associated with increased length of stay, surgical intensive care unit cost, and mortality rate in surgical intensive care unit patients. Feb 9 2012. Am J Surg. 204 (1). 37-43. https://europepmc.org/article/PMC/3992708

[336] A Ginde, J Mansbach, et al. Association between serum 25-hydroxyvitamin D level and upper respiratory tract infection in the Third National Health and Nutrition Examination Survey. Jan 31 2009. Arch Intern Med. 169 (4). 384-390. https://europepmc.org/article/PMC/3447082

[337] L Leow, T Simpson, et al. Vitamin D, innate immunity and outcomes in community acquired pneumonia. Apr 30 2011. Respirology. 16 (4). 611-616. https://onlinelibrary.wiley.com/doi/full/10.1111/j.1440-1843.2011.01924.x

[338] L Muhe, S Lulseged, et al. Case-control study of the role of nutritional rickets in the risk of developing pneumonia in Ethiopian children. May 31 1997. Lancet. 349 (9068). 1801-1804. https://europepmc.org/article/MED/9269215

[339] V Wayse, A Yousafzai, et al. Association of subclinical vitamin D deficiency with severe acute lower respiratory infection in Indian children under 5 years. Mar 31 2004. Eur J Clin Nutr. 58 (4). 563-567. https://www.nature.com/articles/1601845

[340] J McNally, K Menon, et al. The association of vitamin D status with pediatric critical illness. Aug 5 2012. Pediatrics. 130 (3). 429-436. https://europepmc.org/article/MED/22869837

Chapter 12: Religious exemption language

[341] Vaccine Adverse Event Reporting System. US Dept of Health and Human Services. https://vaers.hhs.gov/

[342] Open VAERS. COVID vaccine data. https://openvaers.com/covid-data/mortality

[343] L Le Mahieu. Supreme Court allows CMS vaccine mandate for healthcare workers to go forward. Jan 13 2022. Daily Wire. https://www.dailywire.com/news/supreme-court-allows-cms-vaccine-mandate-for-healthcare-workers-to-go-forward

[344] J Adler. Breaking: SCOTUS stays OSHA vax-or-test rule, allows CMS vaccine mandate for healthcare workers to take effect. Jan 13 2022.   Reason. https://reason.com/volokh/2022/01/13/breaking-scotus-stays-osha-vax-or-test-rule-allows-cms-vaccine-mandate-for-health-care-workers-to-take-effect/

[345] US Equal Employment Opportunity Commission. Fact Sheet: Religious discrimination. https://www.eeoc.gov/laws/guidance/fact-sheet-religious-discrimination

[346] S Perry. Court delivers win to military members denied religious exemptions from Pentagon vaccine mandate. Jan 4 2022. Daily Signal. https://www.dailysignal.com/2022/01/04/court-delivers-win-to-military-members-denied-religious-exemptions-from-pentagon-vaccine-mandate/

[347] L Zhang, A Richards, et al. SARS-CoV-2 RNA reverse-transcribed and integrated into the human genome. Dec 13 2020. Preprint. bioRxiv. https://pubmed.ncbi.nlm.nih.gov/33330870/

Chapter 13: Medical exemption

[348] US Code of Federal Regulations. 45 CFR § 46.116. General requirements for informed consent. https://www.law.cornell.edu/cfr/text/45/46.116

[349] M Martin. Shortages of this at pharmacies may mean longer lines. Oct 26 2021. https://www.eatthis.com/news-shortages-pharmacies-lines/

[350] N Meyersohn. CVS had every advantage, but it lost the pandemic. Here's what happened. Nov 20 2021. CNN Business. https://www.cnn.com/2021/11/20/business/cvs-closings-pharmacy-retail/index.html

[351] CDC. Covid Data Tracker Weekly Review. https://www.cdc.gov/coronavirus/2019-ncov/covid-data/covidview/index.html

[352] T Rogers. The Pan Doctrine is nazi racial hygiene theory version 2.0 with an extra dose of psychosis. Mar 9 2022. https://tobyrogers.substack.com/p/the-pan-doctrine-is-nazi-racial-hygiene

[353] C Farber. Court-ordered Pfizer documents they tried to have sealed for 55 years show 1223 deaths, 158,000 adverse events in 90 days post-release. Dec 5 2021. The Truth Barrier. https://celiafarber.substack.com/p/court-ordered-pfizer-documents-they

Chapter 14: Court cases that have upheld bodily autonomy

[354] C Shattuck. The true meaning of the term "liberty" in those clauses in the federal and state constitutions which protect "life, liberty and property." Mar 15 1891. Harvard Law Review. 4 (8). https://www.jstor.org/stable/1322046

[355] R Standler. Legal right to refuse medical treatment in the USA. 2012. http://www.rbs2.com/rrmt.pdf

[356] C Huber. Catastrophic vaccines: This is not the first. Substack. https://colleenhuber.substack.com/p/catastrophic-vaccines-this-is-not

[357] JT Biggs. Leicester: Sanitation versus vaccination. 1912. P.117, quoted in S Humphries MD, R Bystrianyk. Dissolving Illusions: Disease, Vaccines and the Forgotten History. 2013. https://dissolvingillusions.com

Index

Notes

Notes

Made in the USA
Coppell, TX
21 September 2022

83452127R10128